Foreword

The past three decades have seen impressive advances in development in the East Asia and Pacific (EAP) region. Gains in income and education have been accompanied by reductions in high levels of infant and child mortality and fertility, improved nutritional levels, better hygiene and sanitation, and increased access to health care. Despite these achievements, progress is far from uniform within the region and there are also emerging challenges such as demographic transition, urbanization, adolescent health, tobacco use, and reemerging diseases that are becoming increasingly important. Equally important are the substantial subnational variations in health outcome, especially among the poor. Good health, nutrition, and population (HNP) are critical to breaking the cycle of poverty, poor health, high fertility, and low economic growth.

This EAP Sector Strategy paper is intended to help address the development challenges and policy directions for the World Bank's HNP sector in the region. The EAP sector strategy identifies key lessons learned in the EAP region and presents policy options and recommendations to strengthen the quality and effectiveness of Bank-supported HNP operations. The development of this strategy is closely linked to the Bank's overall sector strategy that identified three major development priorities:

- Improve the health, nutrition and population outcomes of the poor.
- Enhance the performance of health care systems.
- Secure sustainable health care financing.

The World Bank's EAP Sector Strategy for HNP is central to the Bank's mandate to poverty reduction. This regional strategy is not a substitute for country-level strategies; it is meant to provide the guidelines and parameters for use at the country level. Although this paper has been developed primarily for internal use in the World Bank, the successful refinement and implementation of this strategy requires a partnership with individual countries, as well as with other agencies. Thus, the strategy development process is intended to be ongoing and dynamic, continuing to build on best practices and experiences in the region and internationally. This paper is the first step toward that objective. It will continue to evolve as there is consultation with clients and partners in the region.

Eduardo Doryan
Vice President
Human Development Network

Jemal-ud-din Kassum
Vice President
East Asia and Pacific Region

Acknowledgments

The report was prepared by a team of technical specialists in the Health, Nutrition, and Population (HNP) Family of the Human Development (HD) Network of the East Asia and Pacific Region of the World Bank. The work was led by Fadia Saadah, Senior Health and Population Specialist under the guidance of Maureen Law, EAP HNP Sector Manager, and Alan Ruby, EAP HD Sector Director. The HNP team in the EAP region provided important contributions for the development of the paper. James Knowles, Health Economist Consultant, contributed to the development of the paper, Eduard Bos, Population Specialist, prepared the statistical annexes, and Darren Dorkin assisted with portfolio review. Mariam Cleason, Principal Public Health Specialist, Alexander S. Preker, Lead Economist, and James Tulloch, World Health Organization, were the peer reviewers for the paper. Additional comments and guidance on earlier drafts of the report were provided by Tom Merrick, Senior Population Advisor, Susan Stout, Principal Public Health Specialist, and by the regional management team for the EAP region. Patricia Daly assisted with the final revisions of the paper. Chandra Chakravarthi assisted with the document processing.

Executive Summary

Poverty reduction is the World Bank's overarching mandate, and poor health is as much a part of poverty as low income. People living in poverty suffer a disproportionate share of avoidable illness and death largely because of their socioeconomic status. The poor are often trapped in a cycle of ill health exacerbated by the costs of drugs and treatment, hard physical labor, and limited food intake. Good health, population, and nutrition policies are critical to breaking the cycle of poverty and poor health and enabling sustainable economic growth. Good health contributes to improving the overall quality of life and human capital. For example, school learning increases when children are well-nourished. Adequate nutrition allows them to be healthier and more productive adults. Other public health investments such as micronutrient supplementation may forestall the intergenerational transmission of poverty. Moreover, because the poor are more vulnerable to illness and disabling conditions, the economic gains of enabling good health are greater for them.

At the core of the Bank's poverty reduction strategy is the concern that no country can achieve sustainable improvements in economic productivity without healthy, well-nourished, and well-educated people. For this reason, the World Bank has been involved in the HNP sector in the East Asia and Pacific Region through policy advice and dialogue, lending, and analysis. The Bank's level of involvement in different countries varies according to individual country issues and needs. In recent years, the Bank has extended its support to more countries in the region, a trend that is likely to continue.

The main objective of the strategy discussed in this document is to improve the World Bank's effectiveness in HNP in the region. To this end, the challenge is to shape the strategic direction of Bank-supported operations and activities according to sector priorities, while taking into account lessons learned from previous Bank experience in the region. Implementing this strategy will entail a better understanding of the sector's resource constraints and determine how best to allocate the limited resources for maximal effect. Increased selectivity and flexibility will be key to achieving this result.

Several current and emerging issues are common to many of the countries in the region, but equally important is their diversity. Although a regional strategy cannot take the place of a country-specific strategy, the HNP strategy for the EAP region is intended to offer broad guidelines that respond both to the countries' common issues and to their diversity. This regional strategy adheres closely to the Bank's overall HNP strategy and shares the objectives of assisting client countries to:

- Improve health, nutrition and population outcomes of the poor.
- Enhance the performance of health care systems.
- Secure sustainable health care financing.

Strategy development will be ongoing and dynamic, building on best practices and experiences within the region and internationally. This paper is a first step toward that objective. The next steps should be consultation with clients and partners in the region in an ongoing process of sharing and receiving knowledge and information.

Development Challenges

The EAP region has been very successful in reducing previously high levels of child mortality and fertility and improving nutritional levels and in expanding access to health care among previously unserved populations. However, important challenges remain, including:

Unsatisfactory health outcomes, especially for the poor. Despite impressive achievements in many areas, progress is far from uniform within the region. Of most concern, however, are the substantial subnational variations in health outcomes, especially among the poor. These differentials are observed in a wide range of health indicators including: reproductive health, child mortality, malnutrition, and infectious diseases (TB, HIV/AIDS, malaria). These differentials in the region have to be urgently addressed, while at the same time preparing for emerging challenges that are becoming increasingly important (e.g., demographic and epidemiological transition, urbanization, adolescent health, tobacco use, reemerging diseases).

Inequitable and inefficient performance of health systems. The region has relied heavily on government systems which, despite their impressive early gains, are now frequently failing to respond to consumers' demands. But many of these systems are inefficient and inequitable. In addition, the capacity of ministries of health is very limited in the key areas of regulation and quality assurance, consumer education, policy analysis, and monitoring and evaluation. Moreover, the role of the private sector has been growing steadily, but governments in many countries devote relatively little effort to regulating the private sector and certifying its providers. In most countries, the private sector is excluded from public subsidies, which are channeled directly to public health systems through government budgets.

Inadequate health financing. The region spends only 3.0 percent of its GDP on health, compared with 5.5 percent among all middle-income countries. Total health expenditure per capita in absolute terms is similarly low and has declined recently in some of the countries affected by the recent financial crisis. In terms of resource allocation, a high and, in some cases, growing share of limited public health expenditure is channeled to relatively cost-ineffective uses. Sources of financing are about equally distributed between public sources and private out-of-pocket spending. Thus,

addressing the effectiveness of private health spending is important. Many public health systems in the region impose relatively high user fees, especially for inpatient care, and for the poor this can reduce access to needed services and impose catastrophic health care costs on some households. Levels of health insurance coverage are quite low in several countries. Finally, several countries have not yet achieved financial sustainability of previous health improvements.

The Bank's Priorities for the Region

In response to these issues, the HNP strategy identifies three key priority choices for the region. These are:

HNP Priority 1: Improve the health, nutrition, and population outcomes of the poor. The Bank can assist countries in the region, first, by increasing investment in cost-effective public health interventions to improve efficiency and equity of the region's health systems. Second, the Bank can help client countries find out why utilization of health services is inequitable and create appropriate incentives and strategies to address these inequities. Third, policy oversight in intersectoral areas , involving work with other sectors such as education, food and agricultural practices, and transportation, which most affect the health status of the poor will be encouraged and closely monitored.

HNP Priority 2: Enhance the performance of health care systems. First, the regional strategy accords high priority to health promotion and consumer education both to assure that consumers can make informed choices about health care and to increase consumer input into the health system. Second, greater attention will be given to strengthening the policy and regulatory capacity of ministries of health, particularly in such vital areas as regulation and policy control, health promotion and consumer education, policy analysis, and monitoring and evaluation. Third, more Bank support will be targeted to improving the efficiency and equity of government health systems, with particular attention to incentives, pricing, and decentralization. Finally, the strategy calls for mobilizing private sector resources as well as supporting new technologies and approaches to fighting diseases.

ntents

HNP Priority 3: Secure sustainable health care financing. The region's health sector financing needs are expected to grow rapidly. Because public funds are likely to be tighter for some countries, better targeting of resources will be a high priority. That is why the regional strategy accords highest priority to assisting client countries in securing adequate levels of financing. The regional strategy also gives high priority to establishing carefully designed social insurance programs by supporting pilot programs to extend risk pooling.

Implementing the EAP HNP Strategy

Helping the Bank improve the development effectiveness in HNP in the region is the strategy's main objective. The key steps for achieving this are:

- *Increasing selectivity.* Based on the sectoral priorities (identified above) and country-specific needs, the strategy calls for the Bank's work in HNP—both lending and analysis—to be guided by the three HNP priorities. Other criteria for increased selectivity include potential for development effectiveness, resource needs, and rationale for Bank involvement.
- *Addressing country-specific need.* The strategy calls for the development of country-specific strategies for HNP. Maintaining policy dialogue as well as providing operational support for the implementation of key HNP reforms in countries with a significant unfinished HNP agenda is another important element of the strategy.
- *Improving portfolio quality.* The strategy accords high priority to improving quality of the portfolio and putting quality assurance processes in place.

Achieving these objectives will require strengthening monitoring, supervision, and evaluation capacity and enhancing collaboration with governments to address implementation issues of the portfolio.

- *Improving client services.* Improving development effectiveness of the Bank's work also entails enhancement of the Bank's services to clients by: improving clients' access to information and HNP databases; furnishing more user-friendly documentation; providing more responsive lending instruments and processes and a broader range of lending instruments; improving collaboration during project implementation; and seeking feedback from clients regarding Bank performance.
- *Strengthening partnerships.* Effective partnerships with clients, civil society, stakeholders, regional institutions, and other agencies are important elements of the strategy. The strategy calls for strengthening and fostering these partnerships to improve development effectiveness.

The EAP HNP Strategy—An Ongoing and Dynamic Process

The strategy development process will be ongoing and dynamic, building on best practices and experiences in the region and internationally. This paper is a first step toward that objective. The next steps would involve consultation with other partners in the region and internal assessment of the implications of the strategy for the Bank's work in HNP in the EAP. Implementation of the strategy should be monitored closely. This will assist the Bank in strengthening its strategic focus and identifying constraints that may affect the implementation of the strategy.

1 Accomplishments and Development Challenges

The past three decades have seen impressive advances in development in the East Asia and Pacific (EAP) Region. But despite these gains, the health indicators lag behind other development indicators. Moreover, poor health is as much a part of poverty as low income. People who live in poverty suffer a disproportionate share of avoidable illness and death largely because of their socioeconomic status. The poor are often trapped in a cycle of ill health exacerbated by the costs of drugs and treatment, hard physical labor, and limited food intake.

Good health, nutrition, and population (HNP) policies are critical to breaking the cycle of poverty and poor health and to promoting sustainable economic growth in the region. The economic gains of enabling good health are greater for poor people because they are most vulnerable to illness and disabling conditions. Therefore, improving the health of the poor contributes to poverty reduction. Substantial economic growth in the region has contributed significantly to improvements in health. The discussion that follows presents many of these accomplishments in HNP but also examines some of the difficult challenges caused by poor health, malnutrition, and high fertility.

Accomplishments

In recent years countries in the EAP region have reduced their previously high levels of child mortality and fertility and improved nutritional levels. They have also expanded access to health care among previously unserved populations. Compared with other lower and middle-income countries, the EAP region generally has more favorable key health indicators in many areas, including: access to safe water, access to health services, child and adult mortality, maternal health, fertility, and immunization coverage.

Childhood mortality rates for the region have declined substantially in the last few decades (Figure 1-1). For instance, mortality rates among children under 5 years of age (U5MR) have declined from 157 deaths per 1,000 live births in 1970 to 47 deaths per 1,000 live births in 1997. Many countries in the region shared this decline, though at different rates. In Indonesia, for example, U5MR declined from 216 deaths per 1,000 live births in 1960 to 56 deaths per 1,000 live births in 1997; in Vietnam, the corresponding decline has been even more dramatic—from 219 to 45 deaths per 1,000 live births. Many Pacific Islands also experienced a similar decline. In the Solomon Islands, U5MR declined from 99 deaths per 1,000 live births in 1970 to 28 deaths per 1,000 live births in 1997.

East Asia is frequently singled out for its success in reducing fertility rates. During the past 40 years, the region has experienced the most rapid declines in fertility ever recorded (Figure 1-1). In the early 1960s, fertility was above 5 births in all but one country in the region (Japan); in the late 1990s, only one country (Lao PDR) had a total fertility rate (TFR) above 5 births. Excluding China, where fertility is below replacement level, the region's fertility rate is currently 2.7 children.

The EAP region has also succeeded in combating a number of nutritional problems, although its record in this area is still limited. For example, Indonesia has reduced undernutrition (low weight for age) among children under 5 years of age from 40 percent in 1987 to 30 percent in 1998. In China, where an estimated

1

half of the region's iodine-deficient population reside, 83 percent of all salt is now iodized.

Geographic access to health care has improved dramatically in many countries of the region. In Vietnam, for example, 97 percent of the population is within an hour's walk or travel to a health care facility. In Malaysia, the government uses many approaches to increase access to health services, including employing helicopters and boats to deliver health services in some remote areas. In Indonesia, the government has recently deployed a trained midwife in almost every village of the country. Moreover, many countries in the region have made substantial progress in providing access to safe water. Countries where more than 80 percent of the population enjoy access to safe water include: China (83 percent), Republic of Korea (83 percent), Philippines (83 percent), and Thailand (89 percent).

Figure 1-1. Trends in Infant Mortality Rates and Total Fertility Rates, East Asia and Pacific Region

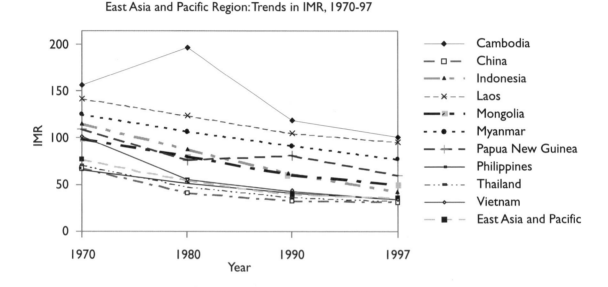

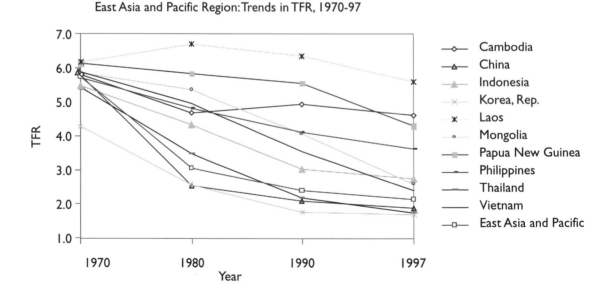

Source: World Bank.

Health programs have certainly contributed to these gains, but it would be incorrect to attribute the region's progress exclusively to this factor. Instead, many factors—including rapid socioeconomic development, political stability, and government leadership—have contributed to the region's health improvements. Economic growth, impressive until recently, has been matched in most cases by progress in female education and in several other social indicators. However, it is easy to overemphasize the role of socioeconomic development. For example, some of the region's most impressive health achievements have occurred in relatively poor Vietnam (relatively high only in education), whereas one of the countries that has performed poorest, the Philippines, enjoys some of the region's highest levels of female education.

Most countries in the region have benefited from a high degree of political stability in recent decades, although some of the most stable countries (e.g., Indonesia) have become less stable since the onset of the region's economic crisis. Other countries in the region (Cambodia, Lao PDR, Myanmar) have experienced warfare and domestic violence during much of the past four decades which undoubtedly has contributed significantly to their relatively poor health performance. Government leadership has also been helpful in supporting selected health, nutrition, and population programs, like family planning and immunization, but has been less effective in other areas, such as tuberculosis (TB) control, maternal health, and health reform.

Development Challenges

Despite impressive achievements in many areas, progress is far from uniform within the region. In some areas, the region's performance as a whole is worse than that of other lower and middle-income countries (i.e., tobacco use, tuberculosis, childhood malnutrition, and anemia among pregnant women). In other areas, individual countries lag behind the region's relatively positive performance (i.e., child mortality, fertility, maternal mortality, malaria, vitamin A and iodine deficiencies). Moreover, some of the earlier achievements are threatened by the recent financial crisis in

the region and its potential negative impact on health outcome.

Of most concern, however, is substantial intranational variation that can still be observed with respect to health outcomes (Figure 1-2). For instance, in Indonesia the U5MR for the poorest quintile in Indonesia is 3.8 times that of the richest quintile; in the Philippines, TFR for the richest quintile is near replacement level while, for the poorest quintile, it remains high at 6.5 births. Other data sources confirm the income gap in health outcomes For instance, information from the Disease Surveillance Points System in China indicates that the infant mortality rate (IMR) among the poorest quartile of the rural population is 3.5 times higher than that among city dwellers. In Indonesia, the prevalence of malnutrition among children in the poorest quintile is 36 percent as compared with 23 percent among children in the best-off quintile.[1]

Key Public Health Areas Currently Affecting the Poor

In addition to those inequalities, health sector performance lags in certain areas within the region. Some of these areas of lagging performance affect most countries of the region (i.e., TB, child malnutrition, anemia, and tobacco use). Other areas are concentrated in a subset of countries. Among the areas that disproportionately affect the poor: are reproductive health, child mortality, malnutrition, and infectious diseases.

Reproductive health. The maternal mortality ratio is above 300 deaths per 100,000 live births in Cambodia, Lao PDR, Myanmar, Indonesia, and Papua New Guinea, and it is above 200 in Thailand and the Philippines. The percentage of births attended by skilled health staff is below 50 percent in Lao PDR, Cambodia, Indonesia, and the Solomon Islands and is below 60 percent in the Philippines, Myanmar, Papua New Guinea, Samoa, and Vanuatu. More than 15 percent of babies born in Cambodia, Lao PDR, Myanmar, Papua New Guinea, and Vietnam are of low birth weight. Tetanus vaccination rates are 60 percent or lower in Indonesia, Lao PDR, Myanmar, Papua New Guinea, and Vietnam. TFR remains above 4.0 births in many countries including Cambodia, Lao PDR, Papua New Guinea, and the Solomon Islands. Additionally,

Figure 1-2. "Under 5" Mortality Rates and Total Fertility Rates, by Income Quintiles: Indonesia, Philippines, and Vietnam, 1997

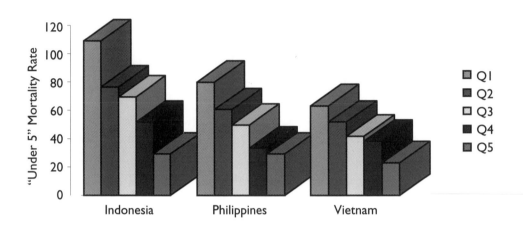

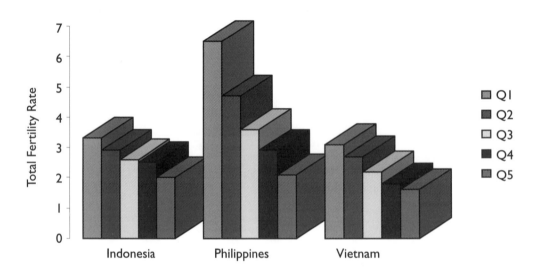

Source: Macro International.

and despite high levels of female education and unmet need, fertility decline has been stalled in the Philippines for many years. Adolescent fertility is above 60 per 1,000 women in Indonesia, Papua New Guinea, and Thailand and above 40 in Lao PDR, Mongolia, and the Philippines.

Child mortality. The U5MR is still above 100 in Cambodia, Laos, and Myanmar. Infant mortality rates for other countries have been stalling. For example, infant mortality rates in China declined by one point

between 1990 and 1997 (from 33 to 32 deaths per 1,000 live births). Moreover, neonatal mortality has declined less rapidly than post-neonatal (1 to 12 months) and child (1 to 4 years) mortality at other ages. In Indonesia, for example, the share of neonatal mortality in total under 5 mortality increased from 29 percent in 1982–87 to 37 percent in 1992–97. This is not surprising, given the high levels of maternal mortality (which is correlated with neonatal mortality) observed in many countries in the region.

Malnutrition. Most countries in the region still have relatively high percentages of children under 5 years with low weight-for-age and height-for-age. Between one-third and one-half of children in Cambodia, Indonesia, Lao PDR, Myanmar, the Philippines, and Vietnam are malnourished by both height-for-age and weight-for-age standards. Improving young children's growth, especially those under 2 years of age, is a high priority for the region. Anemia among pregnant women is another general problem throughout the region. In Indonesia almost two-thirds of pregnant women are moderately anemic.[2] The rate exceeds 50 percent in China, Malaysia, Myanmar, Thailand, and Vietnam and is as high as 45 percent and 48 percent, respectively, in Mongolia and the Philippines. Vitamin A deficiency remains a public health problem in many countries of the region, although some have made progress in recent years in addressing this issue. Moreover, most countries of the region have some areas where iodine deficiency is endemic (Box 1-1).

Infectious diseases. A number of infectious diseases remain important public health problems in the EAP region. TB incidence is relatively high, and resistant strains are rapidly becoming a serious problem throughout the region. The World Health Organization (WHO), in its 1999 report on global TB control, listed 7 EAP countries among the world's top 22 for high TB burdencountries (Box 1-2). TB is projected to cause

Box 1-1. Improved Nutrition Promises Profound Benefits for EAP Region

Good nutrition is the key to healthy development of individuals, families, and societies. But in East Asia and the Pacific, the losses of social productivity are caused by four overlapping types of malnutrition—nutritional stunting and wasting, iron deficiency anemia, iodine deficiency disorders (IDD), and vitamin A deficiencies.

The effects of wasting and stunting are serious for individuals and society. Low birthweight children are more likely to be malnourished. Malnourished children are more likely to die from a common childhood illness, perform less well at school, and grow into smaller adults. Smaller malnourished adults have lower productivity; smaller women are more likely to have low birthweight children. In effect, the problem is intergenerational: malnutrition in one generation contributes to malnutrition in the next. Moreover, malnutrition in early life—including the period of fetal growth—may lead to chronic conditions later in life such as coronary heart disease, diabetes, and high blood pressure. Control of malnutrition has improved somewhat over the last decade, most notably in Thailand, where malnutrition of children under 5 years declined from 51 percent in 1982 to 13 percent at present. But in other countries such as Indonesia, almost 30 percent of children below 5 years of age are malnourished. The challenge for countries in the region is to improve growth in the first 2 years of life by introducing complementary foods with good energy and protein density starting at 4 to 6 months.

Anemia among women and children is a regionwide problem. Although some countries have mounted campaigns to promote iron tablets, compliance has been a continuous problem, and the prevalence of anemia has not been significantly reduced. As recently as 1995, more than 50 percent of pregnant women in Indonesia and Vietnam still suffered from iron deficiency anemia. Current approaches, depending on large-scale campaigns to promote distribution of iron-folate tablets, are not working, and more innovative health promotion strategies are needed, aimed at dietary change and food fortification.

Despite some progress in their control, iodine deficiency disorders and vitamin A deficiency still occur in specific localities and population groups in most countries of the region. Progress has been made in China and Indonesia to universally iodize salt—in China, the coverage of iodized salt is now more than 90 percent in most provinces. The elimination of IDD requires mapping of deficiency areas to allow targeting, distribution of capsules on a short-term basis where deficiency is severe or iodized salt in unavailable, and iodization of salt. Vitamin A deficiency—which causes blindness and damage to the immune system—is still a significant problem in Cambodia, the Philippines, Thailand, and Vietnam. Periodic surveys are needed, allowing targeting of interventions, especially Vitamin A capsules in areas where deficiency is severe, and promotion of dietary interventions where the problem is less acute.

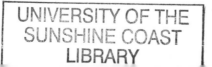

Box 1-2. Tuberculosis, HIV, and Coinfections: Major Public Health Issues

Tuberculosis is a serious public health problem in the EAP region. The World Health Organization (WHO) lists 7 countries—Cambodia, China, Indonesia, Myanmar, Philippines, Thailand, and Vietnam—among the 22 with the world's highest incidence of TB. The TB incidence in most of the EAP region exceeds 100 cases per 100,000 population. The greatest burden of TB morbidity, disability, and mortality is concentrated in adults aged 15 to 59—globally, almost 26 percent of all deaths in this age group are due to TB. Studies have also shown that TB disproportionately affects the lower socioeconomic groups. Prevalence is higher among the undernourished and people living in crowded conditions. And resistant strains of TB are rapidly becoming a serious problem.

HIV is another serious problem in several EAP countries. HIV incidence is still rising in Asia, with more than 1 million new adult infections a year. HIV transmission has moved on from intravenous drug users through commercial sex workers to the general heterosexual transmission . At present, women and children make up close to one-third of all HIV cases in the region, while in Cambodia, Myanmar, and Thailand, approximately 1 to 3 percent of pregnant women are HIV-positive. In contrast, in Indonesia and the Philippines, the disease has remained at the nascent stage.

TB/HIV coinfection, not surprisingly, is a major emerging health issue in this region. The EAP region, along with Sub-Saharan Africa and India, ranks at the top, with coinfection rates of 100 per 100,000 population in Cambodia, Myanmar, Malaysia, and Thailand. By 2020, TB and HIV infection together are expected to account for 92 percent—up from 60 percent in 1990—of adult deaths from infectious diseases. HIV infection, as a risk factor, will account for 25 percent of the TB burden, since lifetime risk of developing TB increases from 5–10 percent to 50 percent in HIV-positive individuals. Inversely, TB occurs in 40–60 percent of those infected with HIV. For these dually infected people, the risk of developing active TB is 30- to 50-fold higher than for people infected with TB alone.

The measures needed to reduce TB morbidity and mortality associated with HIV are much the same as those required to tackle TB alone. This means overcoming the problems that currently limit the effectiveness of TB programs: the inability of many patients to pay for diagnosis and short-course chemotherapy; poor compliance; an inadequate network of reliable laboratories; and an inefficient registration, reporting, and evaluation system for finding new or relapsing cases or assessing treatment results. A number of strategies have been tried out in the region without much success. As for HIV prevention and control, Thailand is the only country in the region that makes a sustained effort to prevent and control HIV. Addressing TB and HIV will require a serious commitment from governments and a strong partnership with the private sector, including nongovernmental organizations.

448,000 deaths in the region in the year 2000. Malaria remains a public health problem in 9 malaria-endemic countries of the region—Cambodia, China (Yunan province), Lao PDR, Malaysia, Papua New Guinea, Philippines, Solomon Islands, Vanuatu, and Vietnam. Malaria incidence in the Solomon Islands remains the highest in the world. HIV/AIDS, prevalent in Cambodia, Myanmar, and Thailand, is rapidly increasing among some groups in China and Vietnam. Deaths from AIDS are projected to increase by almost 90 percent between 2000 and 2010, but then to decline by 22 percent by 2020. Although effective steps to control the spread of the disease have been taken in Thailand, it is raging out of control in neighboring Cambodia.

Care of AIDS patients is a major health sector issue in Thailand.

Emerging Challenges

In addition to the above conditions, where the performance of the region has been lagging, many EAP countries need to take into account new challenges and issues that are increasingly important. These issues are demographic and epidemiological transitions, urbanization, noncommunicable diseases and disabilities, adolescent health, tobacco use, automobile accidents, and reemerging diseases.

Demographic and epidemiological transitions. As the result of its progress in combating infectious diseases and in achieving favorable health and fertility outcomes, the EAP region is going through dramatic demographic and epidemiological transitions. These transitions have important implications for the health sector. For instance, the size of the population in the reproductive age group has been increasing steadily and is projected to keep increasing in the near future (Figure 1-3). This trend has implications for the cost of sustaining family planning and maternal health programs. The size of the elderly population, although still small in most countries, is fast increasing and is becoming more heavily female. These shifts in age and gender composition, success in controlling childhood diseases, and rapid economic growth all contribute both to increases in the overall demand for health services and to an important epidemiological transition in which the share of expensive-to-treat noncommunicable diseases is projected to increase rapidly. As a result of these demographic and epidemiological trends, increases in demand for health care are expected to outpace economic growth.

Urbanization. In addition to changes in age structure, the region's population is becoming increasingly urban (from 39 percent now to 47 percent in 2010).

Although urbanization improves physical access to health services and living standards for some migrants, others will settle in already overcrowded and underserviced slums where they will be even more exposed to certain infectious diseases, pollution, and other environmental risks.

Noncommunicable diseases and disabilities. As noted, noncommunicable diseases (NCDs) are increasingly important in the EAP region. For instance, NCDs accounted for 50 percent of total deaths in the "Other Asia and Islands" Region (burden of disease classification, excluding China) in 1990. This percentage is projected to increase to 75 percent of all deaths in 2020 and will have a large impact on health expenditures unless effective preventive programs are put in place. Disability is another important contributor to the burden of disease, especially in countries that have witnessed widespread conflict. Five of the 10 leading causes of years lived with disability are neuropsychiatric disorders.

Adolescent health is a major neglected problem in many countries of the region. Adolescent fertility is relatively high in Indonesia, Papua New Guinea, and Thailand and, as the data in Figure 1-4 show, is

Figure 1-3. Age and Gender Structure, East Asia Region, 1995 and 2020

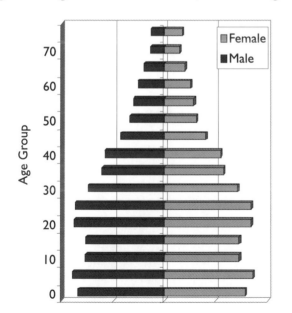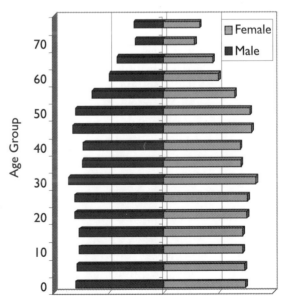

Source: World Bank.

Figure 1-4. Adolescent Fertility Rate by Income Quintile for Indonesia, Philippines, and Vietnam, 1997

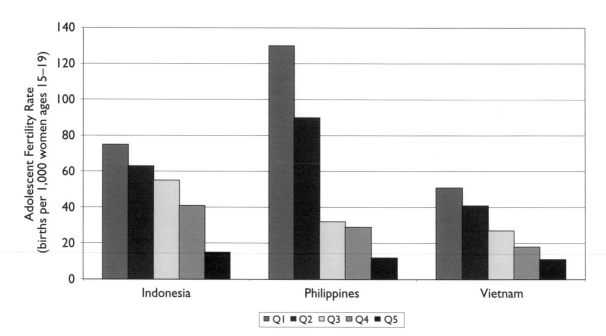

Source: Macro International.

heavily concentrated among the poor. Youths do not even have access to family planning services in several countries. Drug use among youths is reportedly on the rise in Thailand and other countries, particularly since the current financial crisis (driven by relatively high rates of youth unemployment). Youth smoking prevalence is rising rapidly, as are rates of HIV infection in some countries.

Tobacco use. Smoking prevalence is currently 33 percent in population aged 15 or more in the region and growing rapidly. Prevalence among adult males is particularly high (59 percent), compared to only 6 percent among adult females. The available data suggest that smoking is more prevalent among the poor and uneducated. Some governments (e.g., China, Thailand, and Vietnam) have begun to address the problem, but the number of deaths in the region from lung cancer alone is projected to increase by 121 percent between 2000 to 2010, most of them male (Box 1-3).

Automobile accidents (and other injuries) are increasing rapidly in the region. The number of deaths from automobile accidents alone is projected to increase by 54 percent between 2000 and 2020 (from 450,000 to 693,000).

Reemerging diseases and resistant strains of some diseases are an increasing problem in the region. For example, malaria and TB have made a comeback in several countries. Coinfection with TB and HIV is a growing problem (Box 1-2). Resistant strains of malaria, TB, HIV/AIDS, pneumonia, cholera, and dysentery are already common in some countries. In some cases, self-treatment and poor quality treatment exacerbate this problem.

Health System Performance

Most countries in the EAP region have relied heavily on government health systems as the dominant provider of health services. Government services are provided through a multitiered system. At the lowest level, health centers are staffed by one or a few doctors and several paramedics (sometimes supervising a number of health subcenters staffed only by paramedics in rural areas). The next tier consists of district hospitals. Provincial hospitals come next and finally a set of specialist training hospitals. The quality of care, as well as unit costs, increases markedly from the

Box 1-3. Tobacco Epidemic in East Asia and Pacific Region

Smoking now causes 1 in 10 adult deaths. By 2020, 7 of every 10 people killed by smoking will be in low-income and middle-income nations. Of the world's estimated 1,150 million smokers, the EAP accounts for 36 percent. In much of the EAP region, cigarette consumption is rising, and the peak starting age is falling. No longer is there any doubt about the causal connection between tobacco use and chronic disease. Tobacco use also engenders enormous associated costs to society and households globally. For example, smoking-attributed health care costs in China were estimated at 28 billion yuans (about 2 percent of GDP) in 1989.

Some countries, in their strong actions to curb smoking, have increased tobacco taxes to comprise typically around 70 percent of the final selling price. The tax share in cigarette prices in the EAP region varies from 40 percent in China, 33 percent in Malaysia, 36 percent in Vietnam and Indonesia, 62 percent in Thailand, and 63 percent in the Philippines. This suggests potential for raising taxes. This tax increase is expected to slightly reduce cigarette consumption in most countries. Conservative estimates suggest that in China, a 6.5 percent tax increase would be sufficient to finance a package of essential health services for one-third of China's poorest 100 million citizens.

Effective policy options to reduce tobacco consumption include: raising taxes, publishing and disseminating research results on the health effects of tobacco, adding prominent warning labels to cigarette packages, adopting comprehensive bans on advertising and promotion, restricting smoking in workplaces and public places, and widening access to nicotine replacement and other cessation therapies.

Strong action by governments to curb the tobacco epidemic can reduce the terrible economic loss, suffering, and grief from tobacco's burden of disease and premature death. Even modest reductions in a disease burden of such large size would bring highly significant health gains.

lowest to the highest tier. The lowest tier serves mainly rural residents and the poor; the top tier serves mainly urban residents, the rich, and civil servants.

Although most government health systems in the EAP region charge user fees, services are still heavily subsidized. In response to rising incomes, a private health sector has grown up rapidly in most countries, initially providing outpatient services but eventually including private hospital services. The main sources of health care financing in the EAP region are government budgets which are channeled exclusively to the government health system and out-of-pocket financing that pays for user fees in government facilities, private services, and drugs. Consumers' self-treatment of minor illnesses is relatively widespread in the region. Public and private expenditures on health care are fairly evenly divided between government and private financing in most countries. Despite many successes, EAP region government health systems have sometimes failed in areas where they might be expected to excel, and many are less efficient and equitable than consumers have a right to expect.

Consumer knowledge. Traditionally, ministries of health in the region have given low priority to understanding consumer preferences. Many health systems, therefore, do not reflect consumer preferences and needs. Thus, the underutilization of public health facilities commonly observed in the region is not surprising. Moreover, very little emphasis has been placed on consumer education and empowerment. Most consumers in the region are poorly informed about health risks, the benefits of healthy behavior, and ways of making effective choices in health care markets. Although the private sector is successful in attracting clients by providing many of the amenities consumers want (e.g., flexible hours, courtesy, injections, drips), their services vary greatly in terms of quality, are often ineffective (at least, cost-ineffective), and could be wasteful. Many people treat themselves when sick, often purchasing drugs on the advice of inadequately trained pharmacy staff. Such self-treatment and excessive medication have contributed to the development of disease-resistant strains of TB, malaria, sexually transmitted diseases (STDs), and the bacteria that cause pneumonia. Many countries are starting to realize the importance of informed consumers and are focusing much more on health-promotion activities (e.g., the Healthy Indonesia 2010 initiative). However, most of these programs are still concentrating on prevention and promotion and do not go far enough to empower consumers to make informed choices.

Institutional capacity. Government health ministries have usually placed much greater emphasis on their role as service provider than on their role as regulator and policymaker for the entire health sector—public and private. Capacity for effective regulation and quality control, policy analysis, monitoring and evaluation, health promotion, and consumer education is weak in most of the region's health ministries. Extensive information is collected within government health systems, often inefficiently, by vertical programs that collect the same information again and again. However, the information is not broadly disseminated within the system or used effectively by managers to improve the system's performance. Although many of these problems were present and recognized before the recent financial crisis, they became more apparent during the crisis period when a prompt response to the crisis failed to materialize.

Performance of government health systems. Most countries have made dramatic progress in providing their populations with access to basic health services (Cambodia, Lao PDR, and Myanmar are the main exceptions). Physical access to health care is no longer a major problem in the region, although countries such as Indonesia, Thailand, and Vietnam, still have underserviced areas. Performance, however, leaves much to be desired. Most government health systems have performed well when adequately funded and effectively managed. Government health workers are often underpaid and lack incentives to provide their clients with high-quality care. The problem is compounded when the health workers are permitted to have private practices during their off-hours, and by the poor quality of many preservice training programs. These problems undoubtedly contribute to the low utilization of

some types of facilities in several countries. In Indonesia, for example, many health centers are visited by fewer than 50 patients per day, though staffed by 13 or more health workers; and bed-occupancy ratios tend to be low in government class C and D hospitals. The limited success of the health systems has been more pronounced in addressing public health issues that require multisectoral coordination (e.g., HIV/AIDS, malnutrition, malaria in some countries, poor hygiene, environmental health issues).

Decentralization is another challenge facing government health systems . Countries such as China and the Philippines have decentralized their government health systems, and Indonesia has recently initiated a major decentralization process. Decentralization offers many potential advantages (e.g., responsiveness to local needs, accountability, synergy gained from better integration of different programs). However, when it is hurriedly implemented in response to political pressures, health system performance may worsen. In China, for example, decentralization deprived the Epidemic Prevention Service (EPS) of its traditional financing source, the provincial budget. Consequently, it had to rely mainly on user fees, even for services such as TB control. In the Philippines, decentralization has been accompanied by sharply declining immunization and contraceptive use in some regions.

Performance of the private sector. The private sector's role in health care is expanding rapidly in the region. However, in most countries, almost all public subsidies for health care are channeled directly to public health systems through government budgets. Although nongovernmental organizations (NGOs) play an important role in service delivery in some countries (e.g., Pacific Islands), they are not encouraged as service providers in other countries in the region. As a result of such public sector bias in financing, a significant shift occurred from private to public providers in most countries during the recent financial crisis. This shift in demand magnified the negative effects of the crisis for many private providers and placed unnecessary strains on public sector providers at a time when their budgets were being cut.

Governments in many countries devote relatively little effort to regulating the private sector and certifying its providers. As a result, good-quality providers are joined (and to some extent competed out of markets) by poor-quality providers. Traditional healers, though an important source of care in many countries, are typically excluded entirely from government oversight. Consequently, the quality of private care is uneven, and poorly informed consumers face great difficulty in making effective choices.[3] In most countries in the region, private providers sell medications as well as services and tend to overprescribe drugs. Pharmacies staffed by poorly trained personnel and illegal drug vendors routinely sell antibiotics and other prescription drugs freely to the region's consumers.

Health Financing

Resource levels and financing sources. The EAP region as a whole spends 3.0 percent of its GDP on health, compared with 5.5 percent among middle-income countries. Comparable percentages for public spending are 0.8 percent and 3.1 percent. Health spending as a percentage of GDP is particularly low in Indonesia (1.3 percent) and Myanmar (1.4 percent), but it is also low in other countries such as Lao PDR (2.6 percent), and China (2.9 percent). Only in Cambodia is it relatively high (6.9 percent). Health spending has declined from already low levels in most countries as a consequence of the financial crisis. In Indonesia, for example, per capita government health spending declined in real terms in 1997–98 and 1998–99 by 9 percent and 13 percent, respectively. In Thailand, private health spending declined sharply between 1996 and 1998 in real terms. Future growth in health spending, particularly government spending, is likely to be seriously constrained in the aftermath of the financial crisis.

Sources of financing are about equally distributed between public sources (including both the government budget and extra-budgetary social insurance contributions) and private out-of-pocket spending (Table 1-1). The private share of total spending is relatively high in Cambodia (91 percent), Vietnam (91 percent), China (76 percent) and Indonesia (54 percent). Private spending is relatively low in Mongolia (9 percent) and Papua New Guinea (19 percent). Partly because government funding has not kept up with demand, public health systems in the region impose relatively high user fees, especially for inpatient care. High user fees reduce access to needed services on the part of the poor and impose catastrophic health care costs on a subset of households. Such catastrophic costs can have major impacts on household expenditures and may push households below the poverty line.

Resource use. A high and, in some cases, growing, share of limited public health expenditure is channeled to relatively cost-ineffective uses (e.g., curative hospital care for the urban middle class). In Korea, for example, the proportion of the Ministry of Health and Social Affairs' budget directed to primary care declined from 33 percent in 1984 to 11 percent in 1993, while its spending on health insurance subsidies rose from 13 percent of the budget to 44 percent. The share of

Table 1-1. Health Expenditure Financing Sources

	Public (% of GDP)	Private (% of GDP)	Total (% of GDP)
Cambodia	0.6	6.3	6.9
China	0.7	2.2	2.9
Indonesia	0.6	0.7	1.3
Korea	2.5	3.1	5.6
Lao PDR	1.2	1.4	2.6
Malaysia	1.3	1.1	2.4
Mongolia	4.3	0.4	4.7
Myanmar	0.3	1.1	1.4
Papua New Guinea	2.6	0.6	3.2
Philippines	1.7	2.0	3.7
Thailand	1.7	4.5	6.2
Vietnam	0.4	3.9	4.3

Estimates are for most recent year available.
Source: World Bank (see Annex B for details).

China's health budget allocated to preventive care has also declined significantly in recent years while funding increased for the civil servants' health insurance program. In the Philippines the proportion of the central Department of Health budget allocated to public health services declined from 39 percent in 1993 to 29 percent in 1998.

Equity. Partly because government funding has been inadequate, public health systems in the region use relatively high user fees, even for inpatient hospital care. As noted, this reduces use of these services by the poor, imposes catastrophic expenditure on some households, and offers inefficient incentives to providers in some cases. Few efforts in the region have effectively targeted scarce government subsidies to underprivileged and vulnerable groups such as the rural poor and urban slum dwellers. Instead, subsidies are often provided across the board and tend to be relatively large for services consumed mainly by upper income groups (e.g., hospital outpatient services). In Indonesia, for example, government subsidy to health centers (a relatively small share of the total) disproportionately benefits the poorest 20 percent of the population (which receives 24 percent of the subsidy). In contrast, the poor get only 5 percent of the subsidy for hospital inpatient care and only 12 percent of all subsidies, while the richest 20 percent captures 41 percent of the inpatient subsidy and 29 percent of the total. In China, the poorest quartile of the rural population accounted for only 4 percent of all health spending in 1993. The pattern is similar in Vietnam and probably also in most other countries of the region, except Malaysia.

Financing the cost of catastrophic care and risk pooling. Financing the cost of catastrophic care is a major problem in most countries in the region because hospital cost recovery is widely practiced. Levels of health insurance coverage are quite low in several countries (e.g., 18 percent in China, 9 percent in Indonesia, and below 1 percent in Cambodia, Myanmar, and Lao PDR). Although coverage is higher in Thailand and the Philippines, the percentage of health expenditure financed by insurance in both countries remains small (e.g., 4.2 percent of spending in Thailand and 17.6 percent in the Philippines). Any social insurance programs that do exist are usually targeted to select groups such as civil servants or state employees and not to the poor (Figure 1-5). Moreover, most social insurance programs in the region use fee-for-service reimbursement of providers and have done little to control costs. Consequently, consumers are vulnerable to catastrophic costs of health care that could have significant impact on household expenditures. So, when the poor need hospitalization (e.g., for an obstetric emergency), they risk losing their homes or their land. In some cases, this risk deters them from seeking needed care or causes them to delay care until it is too late. Moreover, as a consequence of low social insurance

Figure 1-5. Thailand: Targeting Public Subsidies

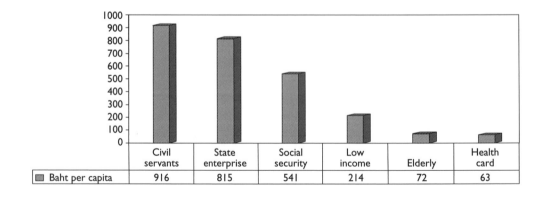

▣ Baht per capita	Civil servants	State enterprise	Social security	Low income	Elderly	Health card
	916	815	541	214	72	63

Source: Prescott, 1998.

coverage, extra-budgetary sources finance a relatively low share of total health expenditure in most countries—less than 20 percent in Indonesia, Malaysia, Philippines, Thailand, and Vietnam; 21 percent in Korea, and 30 percent in China.

Financial sustainability. Several countries have yet to secure financial sustainability of previous health improvements. Many governments have relied on donors to finance family planning and other key public health services and have not made adequate provision to replace donor resources over time. This trend is likely to continue for some time in some of the smaller economies in the region like the Pacific Islands. Additionally, in socialist countries and countries in transition from socialist to market economies, previous sources of funding for health care (e.g., collective farms, state-owned enterprises) have been eroded by market reforms. Although several countries are considering medical savings accounts similar to Singapore's, little progress has yet been made in securing the sustainability of social insurance programs in the face of rapidly aging populations.

ʝic Directions and Policy Options

The countries in the East Asia and Pacific Region are highly diverse in their characteristics. As important as their regional differences and characteristic are, they share many health-related issues and needs. And, these common current and emerging issues offer a place to begin to address the health, nutrition, and population (HNP) status of the region's people. The World Bank's HNP strategy for its work in the EAP region is designed to provide broad guidelines for HNP work that responds both to common issues and to diverse needs. Nevertheless, a regional HNP strategy cannot substitute for country-specific HNP strategies, although the process is similar. Both strategies are devised in consultation with clients, stakeholders, beneficiaries, and other partners, but only country-level strategies can take into account each country's unique needs, past experience, resources, constraints, and opportunities.

This regional strategy adheres closely to the Bank's overall HNP strategy. Both strategies share the following objectives to:

- Improve the health, nutrition, and population outcomes of the poor.
- Enhance the performance of health care systems.
- Secure sustainable health care financing.

These objectives are closely linked because the improvement of health, nutrition, and population outcomes of the poor will require the mobilization of additional resources. Both the amount and the availability of additional resources required depend on the strategy's success in improving the performance of the health care system and in securing sustainable health care financing. Pursuing these objectives in combination can effectively address the problem areas that have limited past health gains among the poor.

Despite commonalities with the Bank's overall HNP strategy, the EAP region HNP strategy focuses on issues that are most important in the region and establishes priorities in some areas. This regional policy will evolve as regional and international experiences and best practice unfold.

Improve the Health, Nutrition, and Population Outcomes of the Poor

According to ample evidence, the poor and other vulnerable groups can significantly improve their health status and general welfare if they increase their use of a basic package of cost-effective clinical and public health services. Investments in such services can, over time, also help to reduce poverty. Improved health among children, for example, increases their productivity in school and allows them to be healthier and more productive adults. Other public health investments may help to forestall the intergenerational transmission of poverty.

This objective of the strategy directly targets several items from the region's unfinished health agenda. Some aspects of the unfinished agenda are visible at the national level (e.g., high levels of maternal mortality, TB, anemia). Others aspects are apparent only upon breaking down data on key indicators by region or income group.

Although the unfinished health agenda is extensive in most countries of the region, examining the magnitude of the problem is not going to be enough to set priorities. The criteria for setting priorities will be based on: the disproportionate effects of the health problem on the poor and other vulnerable groups; the availability of cost-effective interventions to address such health problems; and if the health interventions are associated with market failures or involve public goods.

The main elements of the strategy for improving the poor's health, nutrition, and population outcomes:

- promoting and sustaining cost-effective clinical and public health interventions
- addressing inequities in the utilization of key clinical and public health interventions
- maintaining policy oversight in intersectoral areas that most affect the health status of the poor.

Promoting and Sustaining Cost-Effective Clinical and Public Health Interventions

This strategy emphasizes delivery of cost-effective clinical and public health interventions that address one or more of the health problems that cause the largest burden of disease among the region's poor and other vulnerable groups (e.g., women, children, ethnic minorities). These health problems include malnutrition and micronutrient deficiencies; maternal and perinatal conditions; high fertility rates; and some communicable and vector-borne diseases. Available cost-effective interventions include: immunization, integrated management of childhood illness (IMCI), micronutrient supplements and fortification, health promotion, family planning, and HIV/AIDS prevention.

Many governments in the region have made significant progress in recent decades in making these and other cost-effective interventions available to broad segments of the population. Examples include rapid increases in immunization rates in many countries, family planning gains in Indonesia and Vietnam, iodization of salt in China and Indonesia, and TB and malaria control in Vietnam. However, the share of government health spending directed to these basic public health interventions remains too low. Increased investment in cost-effective public health interventions would improve both the efficiency and equity of the region's health systems. Priority should be given to addressing market failures in such areas as information, externalities, public goods, and intrahousehold allocation. This will promote efficiency and equity by supporting interventions that address the main health problems of the poor and other vulnerable groups. The

priorities for further investment among cost-effective clinical and public health interventions in individual countries should depend on each country's remaining health needs and the degree of success the country has achieved in addressing these needs.

Interventions to address key clinical and public health problems should be efficient, equitable, and sustainable from the outset. Efficiency requires (minimally) that the strategy employed to address a given health problem be cost effective. Governments often tend to scale-up pilot programs before establishing their cost effectiveness. If moving forward quickly is considered urgent, there should still be opportunities for careful evaluation as implementation proceeds.[4] Services also need to be produced efficiently and meet minimum quality standards. Available evidence suggests that some services provided by government health systems do not meet these criteria.

Addressing Inequities in the Utilization of Key Clinical and Public Health Interventions

As noted, many countries in the region have made impressive gains in recent years in providing their populations with physical access to key clinical and public health services. However, the poor and other vulnerable groups do not use these services to the same extent as middle- and upper-income groups. (Table 2-1). Under these conditions, government-supported public health services not only fail the equity test but they also lose their value as poverty reduction interventions. Accordingly, this strategy sets as its highest priority ensuring that the poor and other vulnerable groups utilize cost-effective health services. It also recognizes that achieving this objective may involve major changes in the overall national strategy used to deliver these services.

The first step in addressing this aspect of the unfinished health agenda is to find out why utilization is inequitable. In some cases, the services available to the poor and other vulnerable groups are known to be of poorer quality and less physically accessible. Cultural and linguistic barriers between providers and clients may also impede use in some settings. Lack of incentives among government health workers may result in bad treatment of poor clients in some government health systems. Income and time constraints may pose

...ditional barriers for the poor. The poor also suffer to a greater extent than other groups from lack of information. The main constraints to use of a service by the poor cannot be expected to be the same in all settings. In some cases, constraints may be on the demand side (e.g., education, income, knowledge). In others, they may be mainly on the supply side (e.g., physical access, quality, cost).

Once the main constraints to use have been correctly identified in a particular setting, an appropriate strategy can be developed to increase utilization among the poor and other vulnerable groups. In some countries, the government may have to depart significantly from its national strategy to address the problem. For example, additional incentives may be needed to encourage providers to locate in areas where people are underserved. Contracting with the private sector or nongovernmental organizations (NGOs), may also be considered. In Indonesia, for instance, the Ministry of Health is pilot-testing a strategy of providing vouchers to poor pregnant women that enable them to obtain a basic package of free family planning, safe motherhood, and other maternal and child health (MCH) services from village midwives.

Monitoring success in reducing inequitable utilization requires more detailed information than has been collected in the past. In the future, outcome and service utilization indicators will have to be monitored not only nationally and subnationally but also by income group (and possibly along other dimensions such as gender, religion, and ethnicity).

Maintaining Policy Oversight in Intersectoral Areas

The role of other sectors in improving health outcomes of the poor is also critical and calls for tightening coordination among the health and other sectors. Many sectors' activities affect and are affected by health, and many of the priority areas listed in the first chapter require some level of collaboration with other sectors. These include HIV/AIDS, malnutrition, specific hygiene behaviours, acute respiratory tract infection, adolescent health, and so forth. Among the activities in other sectors with greatest potential impact on the health of the poor are: environmental regulation, water and sanitation programs, basic education and school health programs, and credit programs. In addition, effective coordination with the transport sector may be important in some cases.

Table 2-1. Use of Health Services by Income: Indonesia (1997), Philippines (1998), and Vietnam (1997)

	Income quintiles					
	Q1 (poorest)	*Q2*	*Q3*	*Q4*	*Q5 (Richest)*	*Total*
Measles immunization rate						
Indonesia	59	66	72	75	85	71
Philippines	68	77	83	84	92	79
Vietnam	64	74	82	87	88	77
DPT-3 immunization rate						
Indonesia	52	56	67	66	82	64
Philippines	67	80	84	91	93	81
Vietnam	55	69	64	67	81	66
Pregnant women obtaining two or more antenatal care visits (percent)						
Indonesia	74	88	92	95	98	89
Philippines	76	84	92	93	95	86
Vietnam	33	52	60	72	89	57
Obstetric deliveries attended by a medically trained person (percent)						
Indonesia	21	35	48	64	89	49
Philippines	21	46	73	84	92	56
Vietnam	49	78	84	94	99	77
Contraceptive prevalence rate						
Indonesia	46	56	57	58	57	55
Philippines	20	26	33	33	30	28
Vietnam	47	57	60	80	55	56

Source: Macro International.

Environmental regulation is critical because the poor are often most exposed to the health risks of deteriorating environmental conditions. An estimated 20 percent of the burden of disease in the EAP region results from conditions related to environmental health risks, which predominantly affect the poor and vulnerable groups. Their homes and places of work, for example, are more often exposed to air and water pollution, and they often lack access to safe water and proper sanitation (Table 2-2).

Basic education has been shown to be an important determinant of the health of parents and their children. Fortunately, near-universal primary school enrolment rates in most countries in the region ensure that some basic education is available even to the poor. High levels of school enrollments create opportunities for some cost-effective health sector interventions. For example, public health interventions like health education and iron supplements for adolescent girls can be provided in part by expanding health education in school curricula. However, careful monitoring is needed to ensure that school health programs are equitable, since the children of the poor often do not attend secondary school, or they drop out at an early age.

The poor often find it difficult even to pay for outpatient care and medications obtained from government providers. When seriously ill or injured, often their only option is to forgo needed medical treatment. Improving access of the poor to credit, through microcredit and other programs, can sometimes help the poor gain access to health care. However, access to credit is not enough. Other helpful measures include carefully targeted exemptions from fee payments and free or subsidized health insurance.

Coordinating with the transport sector may also be important where road accidents account for a large share of injuries among the poor. Transportation can also be necessary to ensure access to emergency services (e.g., emergency obstetrical care) among remote rural populations (typically among the most disadvantaged and vulnerable groups).

Enhance the Performance of Health Care Systems

Most countries in the EAP region have previously relied heavily on government health systems to deliver basic health services to all segments of the population. Almost all government financing of health care is currently channeled to government providers. Relying heavily on the direct provision of health services by the government has probably made it easier to secure impressive gains in the provision of relatively simple public health services to large segments of the population. However, it has also presented a number of disadvantages.

The main disadvantage is that ministries of health have been preoccupied with their role as health providers and have largely neglected their role as health regulators, health promoters, consumer educators, and policymakers. Government health systems in countries in the region are too often inefficient and inequitable. A variety of private responses are emerging to deal with consumer demand for more convenient and higher quality services. However, the private sector is inadequately regulated and this, together with

Table 2-2. Access to Safe Water and Sanitation, by Income: Indonesia (1997), Philippines (1998), and Vietnam (1997)

	Income quintiles					
	Q1 (Poorest)	Q2	Q3	Q4	Q5 (Richest)	Total
Households using river, canal, or surface water for drinking (percent)						
Indonesia	48.1	24.5	17.9	7.6	1.4	19.9
Philippines	29.8	11.0	3.8	1.3	0.2	9.2
Vietnam	45.4	18.5	14.3	4.4	1.4	16.8
Households using bush or field as latrine (percent)						
Indonesia	74.3	53.9	41.6	17.9	2.1	38.0
Philippines	-	-	-	-	-	-
Vietnam	53.2	29.7	21.3	12.9	1.7	23.8

Source: Macro International.

˪ᴄᴋ of knowledge of consumers, has led to wasteful consumption of health care.

Measures to enhance the performance of health systems include:

- empowering consumers
- strengthening the policy and regulatory capacity of ministries of health
- improving the efficiency and equity of government health systems
- mobilizing the resources of the private sector
- supporting new technologies and approaches to fighting diseases.

Empowering Consumers

Consumer preferences have been widely neglected in most of the region's health systems, despite the fact that changes in consumer behavior can prevent many serious health problems and consumers in most countries of the regionare responsible for allocating more health sector resources than governments. Smoking, for example, is one of the region 's most serious public health risks. Yet governments have only begun to address the problem through regulation and health promotion. Likewise, HIV/AIDS prevalence is rising rapidly in several countries. Thailand is one of few countries that has adopted effective health promotion measures to address the risks of HIV/AIDS infection. Although injuries from traffic accidents are increasing rapidly, health promotion in this area is weak or nonexistent. Few countries in the region have actively promoted healthy diets and exercise, despite a substantial and growing body of research that demonstrates that both are effective in preventing many noncommunicable diseases. The regional strategy accords high priority to such cost-effective health promotion interventions.

Although private providers of modern medical care have developed rapidly alongside traditional providers in most countries, consumer capacity to make informed choices from among the many available providers has not kept up with the development of private health care markets. Household expenditure on health care typically accounts for one half or more of total health care spending in the region. Yet, much private health care expenditure is channeled to ineffective

or unnecessarily expensive forms of care. Broad consumer education and health promotion designed to equip consumers with the information to make more cost-effective choices in private health care markets should be supported. Consumer education in this area can be particularly effective if combined with strong licensing and certification programs and with effective enforcement of regulations against the uncontrolled dispensing of prescription drugs.

Although the region's governments need to increase their emphasis on health promotion and consumer education, the flow of information should not be in only one direction. Government health systems urgently need feedback from consumers about their satisfaction with the services they obtain. Systematic consumer feedback, especially from the poor and other vulnerable groups, should be an integral part of any quality assurance program. Consumer feedback and inputs are also vital elements in any process of reforming or changing the health system. In some settings, community participation in the health sector has been institutionalized through community health committees or health boards. It is particularly important to ensure that the poor and other vulnerable groups are adequately represented in such community health organizations.

Strengthening the Policy and Regulatory Capacity of Ministries of Health

Many ministries of health in the region have focused almost exclusively on developing their service delivery capacity and have failed to develop capacity in such vital areas as regulation and quality control, health promotion and consumer education, policy analysis, and monitoring and evaluation. This strategy places high priority on strengthening capacity in these areas. However, this does not mean that all capacity has to be developed in-house. Among the capacities that need strengthening most urgently, only the regulatory function cannot be contracted out to universities and NGOs. Quality control, including licensing and certification, can be largely delegated to professional organizations. Health promotion and consumer education activities could also be contracted out. Evaluation research and policy analysis can be contracted out to universities and other research organizations. However, a certain level of capacity is needed even in these areas within ministries to manage the activities of external collaborators, to extract the most relevant findings from their work, and to communicate them effectively to other units within the ministry.

The regulatory and quality control area needs much development and improvement within the region. These activities should cover both the public and the private sectors. However, conflicts of interest may arise when ministries of health attempt to regulate the private sector while operating competing operations in the public sector. For example, in pharmaceutical manufacturing and distribution, the government must implement strict quality control. Counterfeit drugs and illicit drug distribution are common in the region. However, government's frequent involvement in both the manufacture and distribution of pharmaceuticals could present a conflict of interest. Another danger is that the privatesector groups to be regulated will "capture" the regulatory process. Often this is manifested in ministries' efforts to limit competition within the private sector. In fact, in many countries in the region, the best developed aspect of government health sector regulation involves regulations designed to restrict competition.

Effective enforcement of regulations and quality controls is needed: regulations are necessary but not sufficient. Effective regulation and enforcement is greatly facilitated when the regulatory process involves the active participation of consumers and providers. Corruption is also a problem in some government health systems, and most commonly affected is the procurement of pharmaceuticals. Although improvements in this area are most likely to come as part of a general strengthening of governance within the region, pharmaceutical reform within the health sector (e.g., essential drug lists) can also contribute to this objective.

One important area of government involvement in the health sector that has been largely neglected is the supply of information to consumers. As discussed, increased government effort is needed both in the areas of health promotion and in educating consumers to make better choices in private health care markets. Governments are unlikely to be efficient producers and disseminators of such information. However, they need to establish priorities among the many health messages that can be communicated, subsidize the production and dissemination of these messages, monitor and evaluate their effectiveness, and restrict harmful and misleading advertising.

Many ministries of health in the region lack effective policy analysis units. As the private sector develops and especially as steps are taken to extend risk-pooling services to a larger share of the population, the capacity to do good-quality policy analysis must be developed within a ministry of health. Some of the needed expertise can be obtained from universities and other research institutes, as is done effectively in the Philippines and Thailand. But ministries need a core policy analysis capability of their own to manage the necessary analyses and to communicate their findings effectively.

Monitoring and evaluation is another important function for which little capacity has yet been developed in most ministries of health. Particularly in a decentralized health system—as recent experience in the Philippines has demonstrated—ministries need to carefully monitor certain key health indicators not only at national and regional levels but also among the poor and other vulnerable groups. Many countries do not have adequate information systems or regular surveys to measure health indicators. Monitoring efforts should also focus on the efficiency of resource utilization at the local level as well as whether the allocation of resources within local areas is equitable. At the national level, national health accounts can be useful tools for monitoring progress in health financing and in use of key services by the poor and other vulnerable groups.

Improving the Efficiency and Equity of Government Health Services

Ministries of health in most countries manage large and diversified service delivery organizations. Some government health systems have been effective and reasonably efficient in providing the entire population with access to basic health services (Malaysia). When effective, government health systems have been well funded and have adequately compensated their staff, including extra compensation for working in less desirable locations. Government providers in those systems have not felt they had to develop private practices on the side, and they have been motivated to provide good-quality services. Effective government health systems have also found ways to decentralize management functions to lower levels of government and to delegate more authority to facility managers.

Unfortunately, government health systems in many countries in the region do not exhibit these positive features. Since most governments in the region are likely to continue their role as providers of health services, an important part of the regional strategy involves identifying ways to improve the quality and efficiency of government health services. The three most likely areas are: incentives, pricing, and decentralization.

Inadequate incentives are an important cause of inefficiency in government health systems. Budgets are often allocated to facilities on the basis of facility size instead of volume of services provided. Staff members are typically underpaid and are often permitted to supplement their income through private practice outside normal working hours. Supervision is typically weak, again due in part to the absence of incentives. Rewards are few for those who perform well. Training is often either ineffective or unsustainable because after training people have no incentive to use what they learn.

The challenge is to find a way to strengthen appropriate incentives within a government health system. One effective approach is to improve compensation levels generally, strengthen supervision and staff evaluation, and build in systems to reward staff for good performance. When this is done, private practice outside normal hours and accepting side payments can be resisted.[5] The problem is that implementing this strategy sometimes requires broad civil service reforms. Additionally, facilities can be permitted to charge limited fees for services and to retain the revenue for quality improvement and staff incentives. However, most countries in the region have already introduced user fees for a broad range of health services, and raising them would risk further restricting the use of services by the poor and other vulnerable groups.

Another approach would be to stimulate increased efficiency within the government health system by promoting competition between it and private providers. Although government health systems in the region already compete in a broad sense with the private sector, they rarely compete for the same clients. The private sector tends to serve middle- and upper-income clients, while the government health system serves mainly the lower income groups. However, government often serves its segment poorly. Targeted demand-side financing of services for the poor could offer government providers a powerful incentive to improve care to poor clients. This could simultaneously raise service utilization rates among vulnerable groups and improve the efficiency and equity of government health systems.

Current pricing policies in government health systems contribute significantly to the patterns of inefficiency and inequity observed in many countries (i.e., underutilization of primary care facilities, low shares of government subsidies captured by the poor). The pricing of hospital outpatient services is particularly problematic. These services tend to be used mainly by middle- and upper income urban residents. As a general rule, fees charged for hospital outpatient care should be equal to their marginal social cost. If such facilities provide public health services , the absolute subsidy should be no greater than the subsidy provided for the same services in primary care facilities. Current hospital outpatient care pricing practices within the region depart significantly from this model. Although the fees charged are typically much higher than those fees at primary care facilities, the absolute unit subsidy is typically much greater for hospital outpatient services than for the same services obtained from primary care facilities. This pricing policy provides a powerful incentive to consumers to use these facilities unnecessarily and is responsible for much of the inequitable distribution of benefits within government health systems. The pricing of inpatient care is a special case. Until insurance coverage is universal, a strong case can be made for subsidized prices on the grounds of risk pooling. However, subsidies must be better targeted to benefit the poor and vulnerable groups.

Decentralization can result in more efficient government health systems if the services can be made more responsive to local needs without compromising other dimensions of efficiency or equity. However, if decentralization is to improve the efficiency of government health systems, careful preparation is necessary.

When central governments simply download responsibilities for managing health facilities to local governments without careful preparation, performance is likely to suffer and the system may even become more inefficient than before.[6] Careful preparation includes deciding which functions should be devolved and to which level of authority. Some functions involve substantial economies of scale and should not be devolved to local governments. Other functions involve externalities beyond local areas (e.g., immunization, disease surveillance) that require proper incentives to ensure that socially efficient levels of services continue. Some functions such as auditing, monitoring, and evaluation may need to be retained and strengthened at the central level. Also, local government staff must be adequately trained to manage the facilities within their jurisdiction. Furthermore, careful preparation for decentralization includes ensuring that local resources are sufficient to operate and maintain devolved facilities. In this regard, effective mechanisms need to be in place to transfer resources from the central government to relatively poor local governments. Finally, decentralization of the health sector must be understood in light of the decentralization of public administration across other key related sectors.

Mobilizing the Resources of the Private Sector

Although countries face genuine options in selecting an appropriate mix of public and private financing of health care, the relative importance of private provision is likely to grow rapidly as countries develop. Such a trend is expected because private providers may be able deliver the same services at lower cost and offer a wider range of quality and other features that consumers demand as their incomes rise. The fact that even Malaysia, where the government health sector has been effective, has already begun to evaluate a wide range of privatization options suggests that such a trend is unavoidable.

Despite the apparent success of the private sector in responding to consumer demand, private health providers (and private insurers) require effective government regulation and other public interventions if health market outcomes are to be efficient and equitable. The strategy also calls for the selective use of demand-side financing and performance-based contracting to mobilize the resources of the private sector (including NGOs) to serve the poor more effectively than public systems have been able to do.

Although the strategy recognizes that some government health systems in the region are likely to be continue to provide services in the near future, countries that as yet have undeveloped government health service delivery systems may wish to explore other options for investing their relatively limited resources. While a case can be made for government investment in developing a basic primary care infrastructure in currently underserved rural areas, why the curative care activities of such a system must always be managed by the government is unclear. Governments can examine alternative mechanisms to deliver services through contractual arrangements with NGOs and private providers. Moreover, experience in many countries, within and outside the region, indicates that even low-income consumers prefer private outpatient care.

This strategy does not support the expansion of private health insurance (for reasons discussed more fully below). However, it strongly supports the integration of private providers into social health insurance programs. The argument that social insurance programs cannot afford to extend benefits to include services obtained from private providers because they are more "expensive" than those of public providers usually fails to consider the full cost of government services. The main value of insurance over subsidized direct provision of health care by the government is the opportunity it affords for increased competition in health care markets. Including private providers in social insurance programs necessitates effective cost controls, but experience in China and Vietnam suggests that these are desirable even when benefits are limited to services obtained from government providers.

Supporting New Technologies and Approaches to Fighting Diseases

New technologies and service delivery approaches (e.g., integrated management of childhood illness, vaccination against hepatitis B) are under continual development and evaluation to combat various public health threats. Further innovations are possible not only in the areas of prevention, diagnosis, and treatment (e.g., HIV vaccines, malaria diagnosis, HIV therapy) but also in the organization, delivery, and management of health systems (e.g., computerized information systems at the facility level, supported by advanced communications) and in the training of health manpower (e.g., distance learning). There may be similar opportunities for transferring methods developed in other regions for reorganizing or financing health services. After careful evaluation, many of these innovations may be introduced to the health care market in the EAP countries. To this end, the Bank has a comparative advantage in scaling-up these new technologies and approaches in its sector lending. In some cases, questions may still be unanswered about how well these new methods will perform when scaled up in actual health systems. In such cases, the Bank can work with other partners to carefully evaluate their performance either beforehand or as the scaling-up process proceeds to ensure that they are cost effective.

Secure Sustainable Health Care Financing

This objective—securing sustainable health care financing—addresses the region's health sector financing needs, which are projected to grow rapidly. Moreover, and in view of the recent financial crisis in this region, public funds are likely to be more constrained, and better targeting of these scarce resources is a high priority for many countries in the region. The region also needs to expand risk-pooling services, which are relatively underdeveloped at present.

Securing Adequate Levels of Financing

Currently, most lower and middle-income countries and their governments in the EAP region probably underspend on health. The main sources of health sector financing currently are private out-of-pocket spending by households and government financing. Extra-budgetary financing is still limited in most countries. It accounts for only 9 percent of health expenditure in Thailand, 11 percent in Indonesia, and 12 percent in the Philippines, compared with 30 percent in China and 21 percent in Korea. Over time, with current demographic and epidemiological trends, it will be increasingly difficult for government financing to

keep up with rapidly growing demand for health care, even assuming continued progress in fiscal reform and successful efforts to promote healthy practices on the part of consumers. Diversification of financing beyond the government budget is probably the key to expanding the resources available to the health sector. The expansion of extra-budgetary financing through mandatory social insurance is the most promising approach to increasing the level of health sector financing in the long term. Other possible sources of financing are private households and central and local governments.

Private households. Out-of-pocket spending by households is currently the main source of health service financing in most countries of the region, and it is not limited to private outpatient providers as it usually is in other regions. In Indonesia, for example, one quarter of out-of-pocket spending is directed to government providers, half of it to government hospitals. Out-of-pocket financing is not an equitable source of financing. The poor have very limited resources to devote to health care, so excessive reliance on out-of-pocket financing leads to an inequitable distribution of health care. In addition, the heaviest burden of out-of-pocket expenditures falls on the least healthy who are therefore less able to shoulder this additional burden. User fees are already widely used in government health systems in most countries in the region, and evidence indicates that they already restrict access of the poor to services. This strategy, for most countries, calls for a reduction in reliance on out-of-pocket financing as a source of financing for inpatient care and, particularly, in the share of out-of-pocket financing borne by the poor.

Governments. A strong case can be made that governments should expand their commitment of resources to the health sector. The highest priority for the use of additional resources should be to raise the utilization of key public health services by the poor. However, since the region's financial crisis, many governments face serious short- and medium-term fiscal constraints on their ability to increase spending. Fortunately, most governments in the region have some scope to reallocate health sector subsidies from less efficient and equitable services to critical public health services that will benefit the poor. For example, reducing high unit subsidies to hospital outpatient services would reduce the share of total subsidies that go to the rich and encourage higher income consumers to use lower cost primary health providers for routine outpatient care.

Some forms of decentralization create the possibility of mobilizing additional resources for the health sector at the local level. Where local authorities retain and allocate at least some locally generated tax revenue, communities may be willing to pay higher taxes to improve the quantity and quality of available health services. In some settings, local governments have also been able to mobilize additional taxes to support community risk-pooling programs. The main problem with resource mobilization at the local level is that local taxes tend to be inefficient and inequitable. Relying too heavily on locally generated resources can also lead to geographical inequities, since relatively wealthy localities can more easily raise additional resources than poor communities. This became a problem in Vietnam when commune health centers were financed mostly at the commune level.[7] Locally administered risk-pooling programs also tend to have relatively high administrative costs (e.g., dana sehat in Indonesia).

Expanding Access to Risk Pooling Through Social Health Insurance

It is the nature of health care spending to become concentrated in a small proportion of the population. Although a minority of the population incurs catastrophic health care expenses at any one time, any one may face the risk of such costs at some time in life. Most people are willing to pay to convert this risk, through insurance, into a more predictable and manageable periodic outlay, based on average health care costs among a large pool of consumers.

Traditionally, risk-pooling services have been provided in the region through highly subsidized government health systems. However, the inability of government funding to keep up with fast-growing demand for increasingly expensive health care in many countries has expanded the role of out-of-pocket financing for health services, including relatively expensive inpatient care in government hospitals. The poor, most often lacking savings and access to credit, have trouble financing even routine outpatient care in primary

health facilities and either have to look to family and friends for assistance, sell their few assets, or do without needed health care.

Ordinarily, unmet demand for risk-pooling services could be satisfied through private insurance, but markets for private health insurance do not operate normally. Consumers are better judges of their individual health risks than insurers. The resulting client "selectivity" means that the insured pool has much higher average health care costs than the general population. The problem of selectivity (as well as the problem of collecting premium payments) can be avoided if insurers sell coverage to a group formed for some purpose other than to purchase insurance. The employees of a large firm constitute such a group, and private health insurance is usually marketed to groups of employees. However, in many EAP countries opportunities to form risk pools are few since most of the labor force is still engaged in agriculture or informal sector work.

These conditions severely limit the potential for private, voluntary health insurance.[8] Although the demand for private insurance can be expected to grow as the size of the formal sector expands, it is unlikely ever to provide risk-pooling services for the people who need them most, namely the poor. Instead, private insurers tend to recruit better-off and healthier consumers to whom they can afford to offer generous policies at reasonable cost. Higher utilization by the insured compounds inequity within the health system, contributes to cost escalation, and creates a powerful constituency opposed to the development of broader social health insurance.

The risk-pooling needs of the general population can be most practically met by encouraging the systematic expansion of mandatory social health insurance coverage to successively higher proportions of the population—and ultimately to the entire population. Most governments in the region are actively developing and testing ways to extend social health insurance coverage to previously uncovered groups. Coverage has been expanding steadily. In Thailand, the government recently decided to expand social health insurance coverage(previously limited to government workers) to employees of large private firms. In Indonesia, the government is supporting expanded coverage of managed care (JPKM) to previously uncovered groups.

The task of extending social health insurance coverage to rural populations and to those workers in the urban informal sector is particularly challenging because of difficulties in forming risk pools and in collecting premiums.[9] However, poverty is concentrated in these groups; and the welfare impact on the poor of catastrophic medical expenses is commensurately greater. Accordingly, the regional strategy gives high priority to supporting innovative pilot programs, designed to extend risk pooling to agricultural and informal sector workers as well as to scaling up successful approaches.

In the process of becoming universal, there is a risk that social health insurance will make health systems more inequitable. This problem arises because utilization rates of the insured tend to be higher than those of the uninsured and because they have higher incomes than the uninsured. Inequity is compounded if the services used by the insured are heavily subsidized. Social insurance programs could circumvent this problem by reimbursing government providers for the full cost of services, not just for user fees. Such a policy also opens up the possibility for private providers to compete fairly with government providers.

Cost control is another key issue that needs to be addressed in the early stages of a social health insurance program. Cost control has been a serious problem, for example, even in the early stages of Vietnam's health insurance program. If social health insurance programs rely upon fee-for-service payments, as they do in most countries in the region, introducing cost controls (e.g., coinsurance, copayments, and deductibles) should be a high priority. These devices also help to control inequities in use between the insured and uninsured while coverage is being expanded.

"First-dollar" coverage (instead of coverage for catastrophic care) presents another problem under some EAP countries' social insurance programs (e.g., Thailand and the Philippines). This means that these programs do not secure the full benefits of risk pooling. At the same time, generous coverage for routine expenses (e.g., drugs in connection with outpatient care) can lead to excessive consumption of these items by the insured. The appropriate policy is to limit social health insurance coverage initially to catastrophic care and gradually deepen benefits as coverage and incomes rise (and as administrative capacity to control costs develops).

Carefully designed social health insurance programs can effectively address horizontal risk-pooling needs. However, as populations age, the financing burden on the working population can become very heavy (as many European countries have found). Countries could consider programs like the medical savings accounts, developed in Singapore to prepare for the growing cost of providing medical care to aging populations.[10] can also make more stringent cost controls possible, but, as with all deferred benefit programs, people have to believe in the financial integrity of the institutions managing these funds. Mandatory savings plans are also difficult to implement when most people work in agriculture and the informal sector. Consequently, not every country in the EAP region is ready for broad-based medical savings account plans.

Conclusions

This chapter has identified the following priorities and strategic direction for the HNP work in the region:

- *Improve the health, nutrition, and population outcomes of the poor* by promoting and sustaining cost-effective public health interventions; addressing inequities in the use of key public health interventions; and maintaining policy oversight in intersectoral areas that most affect the health status of the poor.
- *Enhance the performance of health care systems* by empowering consumers; strengthening the policy and regulatory capacity of ministries of health; improving the efficiency and equity of government health systems; mobilizing the resources of the private sector; and supporting new technologies and approaches to fighting diseases.
- *Secure sustainable health care financing* by securing adequate levels of financing; and expanding access to risk pooling through social health insurance.

3 The World Bank's Role in HNP: Strengthening Our Development Effectiveness

The first two chapters outlined the key development challenges and policy directions for the health, nutrition, and population (HNP) sector in East Asia and Pacific Region. This chapter deals with the implementation of this strategy and its implications for the Bank's work in the EAP region. Strategy development is an ongoing and dynamic process, building on best practices and experiences in the region and internationally. These recommendations are the first step toward this objective. Consultation with clients and partners in the region and consideration of experiences and best practices in the sector will further enhance the strategy development work. Such a vision of the strategy would also enhance knowledge-sharing with client countries and other partners.

The World Bank Role in HNP

Investments in health, nutrition, and population are essential parts of poverty reduction efforts and a key to sustainable economic growth in the region. Improving health improves productivity. It permits the use of natural resources that had been totally or nearly inaccessible because of disease, raises school enrolment and educational attainment, and frees resources that would have been spent on treating illness for alternative uses. The economic gains are greater for poor people who are usually more affected by ill health.

Over the past three decades, the Bank has been an important player in the HNP sector in the region through policy advice and dialogue, lending, and analysis. The Bank's involvement in the different countries varies significantly, a reflection of the large diversity of issues and needs across the region. Since the early 1970s, the Bank has financed HNP programs in 10 countries for a total of $2.2 billion. Most of the Bank financing has been concentrated in China (37 percent) and Indonesia (33 percent). In recent years, the Bank has expanded its support to more countries in the region and is likely to be involved in even more countries in the near future (e.g., Samoa and Myanmar). The HNP portfolio has grown significantly over the years, especially between 1991 and 1996. However, the last three years (fiscal years 1997–99) saw a decline in the volume of investment lending for this sector. This decline may be partially due to the East Asia financial crisis as well as the graduation of some client countries to IBRD lending terms (e.g., Philippines).

At present the EAP human development unit (EASHD) manages 22 operations with a total lending volume of $1.3 billion. Nearly three-fourths of the lending volume is in China (47 percent) and Indonesia (26 percent). The distribution of the lending program is especially significant, considering that the future of the lending program in China is uncertain since its graduation from IDA borrowing terms in July 1999. In terms of focus, the projects cover a wide range of issues, depending on the country characteristics (Annex C). In general, the Bank supports more "hard ware" components in the region's less developed countries that are still building their health systems. However, the Bank's role has been evolving in other countries, financing projects to improve the performance of existing health systems and addressing priority health problems. Through the current emphasis on dealing with health system issues, the Bank is attempting to address some of the underlying constraints that limited the effectiveness of earlier efforts. China, Indonesia, the Philippines, and Vietnam fit into this category. As discussed in Chapter 2, many EAP countries face more difficult policy choices including issues of health system performance (both public and private sectors), empowering consumers, health-financing options, and so forth. In response, some countries are likely to need assistance that goes beyond the scope of the current program.

Evaluating the Bank's lending HNP performance in the EAP region is not easy. One way would be to look at project ratings. The percentage of projects rated satisfactory has improved over the years, but this trend reversed during the financial crisis along with the performance of many investment operations. Moreover, some useful insights about the HNP portfolio in EAP can be drawn from the recently completed worldwide study by the Operations Evaluation Department of the Bank's HNP operations (*Investing in Health: Development Effectiveness in the Health, Nutrition, and Population Sector*). This study concludes that Bank investments have provided valuable support in expanding and strengthening the building blocks of public health systems (e.g., facilities, staff). The benefits of these investments have been hindered by continued systemic problems in the delivery system and by poor quality and underfunding of basic services. The study also concludes that the performance of the client countries and the country context are the two most important factors in project performance. As for the factors the Bank can influence, the three most important are assessment of borrower institutions and capacity, strong supervision, and attention to monitoring and evaluation. These conclusions are applicable and relevant to the experience of the HNP sector in the EAP region.

Analytic and advisory services (AAA) are another important part of the Bank's work in HNP. Analytic work is key for policy dialogue and should provide the needed diagnostics for the lending operations. The region has supported AAA activities that influenced or facilitated important policy changes; assisted in capac-

ity-building efforts; and provided the background and analytic basis for important lending operations. The Bank is supporting two strategy development exercises in Vietnam and Indonesia. Despite these important contributions, the linkages between AAA activities and lending operations must be strengthened, and effectiveness of such effort and responsiveness to sector needs must be ensured.

Country assistance strategies (CAS) are another useful tool for addressing HNP issues as part of a country's overall development framework. The EAP region has been generally successful in ensuring that HNP issues are highlighted in most CAS exercises. However, the linkages of HNP issues with the macroeconomic analyses and poverty alleviation strategies could be strengthened. Moreover, multisectoral issues are not generally given adequate attention during the CAS exercise. The comprehensive development framework (CDF) could provide an opportunity for addressing these issues.

How does the current portfolio fit with the proposed strategy? Although the current activities are consistent with the proposed strategy, many priority areas have been given little attention. These include health financing, performance of the private sector, consumer empowerment, and cross-sectoral efforts. Even in areas the portfolio addresses—like health outcomes of the poor—many gaps in our knowledge and coverage of these issues remain. Implementing the proposed strategy is going to require more selective but intensive efforts to respond to the priorities as they relate to the different country programs.

Implementing the World Bank's EAP Regional HNP Strategy

The main objective of the strategy is to improve the Bank's development effectiveness in HNP in the region. To this end, the challenge for the HNP sector is how to shape the strategic direction of Bank–supported operations and activities in line with sector priorities identified earlier, while taking into account the lessons learned from previous Bank experience in the sector in the EAP region. Implementing the strategy entails considering the resource constraints facing the sector and the best ways of allocating limited resources to maximize the development impact of the operations. Increased selectivity and flexibility will be key to achieving this result and to making the most of the available resources.

Sharpening Strategic Direction

The first step toward implementing the strategy involves sharpening the strategic direction of the World Bank–supported activities in line with priorities identified in Chapter 2. These priorities are:

HNP Priority 1. Improve the health, nutrition, and population outcomes of the poor by:
* promoting and sustaining cost-effective basic clinical and public health interventions
* addressing inequities in the use of key public health interventions
* maintaining policy oversight in intersectoral areas that most affect the health status of the poor.

HNP Priority 2. Enhance the performance of health care systems by:
* empowering consumers
* strengthening the policy and regulatory capacity of ministries of health
* improving the efficiency and equity of government health systems
* mobilizing private sector resources
* supporting new technologies and approaches to fighting diseases.

HNP Priority 3. Secure sustainable health care financing by:
* securing adequate financing
* expanding access to risk pooling through social health insurance.

Increased Selectivity

The strategic direction outlined above is necessary but not sufficient for the Bank to set priorities in terms of lending operations and AAA. To achieve greater selectivity in the HNP work program across countries, as well as within countries, potential for development effectiveness, resource needs constraints, and rationale for Bank involvement should also be considered when selecting activities for Bank support.

* *Potential for development effectiveness.* Development effectiveness of Bank–supported activities should be a key criterion for setting priorities. Despite the variations in method for measuring development effectiveness of specific operations, some key determinants of development effectiveness must be taken into account. For instance, past experience shows that development effectiveness of lending operations depends on the general policy framework (including institutional effectiveness) for the sector. Thus, lending operations should be evaluated against such a framework. In fact, if the policy framework is such that development impact is unlikely, then Bank involvement may be limited to selected analytic work such as program monitoring and to establishing contact or continuing dialogue. Country factors and context are also key factors affecting the ability of Bank operations in HNP to achieve their development objectives. Strong demand and ownership by the client country for achieving development impact should be considered a prerequisite for successful operations. Likewise, AAA activities must be assigned priority in light of their potential development impact. The approach may be different, however, and will depend on the likely effect of the analysis on the sector in a specific country, at regional level, and beyond.
* *Resource needs constraints.* Because resources are limited, an operation's resource requirements must be weighed against its potential development impact. Analysis of resource requirements should not be limited to preparing lending operations but should also cover project supervision. Such an analysis will require planning for resource allocations beyond annual allocations.
* *Rationale for Bank involvement.* The issues affecting the health sector in the region are numerous. Whether the Bank is the "best" choice to address these issues depends, in part, on the rationale for government involvement, on the likely effectiveness of Bank–supported operations to address the sector issues, and on the role of other partners.

Addressing Country-Specific Needs

Diversity is one of the region's main features. To the extent permitted by available information, grouping the countries by characteristics would perhaps be useful, for example, by economic development, health outcomes (especially of the poor), performance of the health care system (Box 3-1); and health financing profile. Clusters of countries could then be examined by the products they are likely to seek from the Bank.

The first set of countries has good health outcomes, good economic indicators, and well-developed health care systems: Hong Kong, Singapore, and South Korea. These countries do not normally borrow for the HNP sector but are a rich resource for the region and important partners for the Bank, especially in analytic and advisory activities. The strategy calls for their increased participation in the generation and dissemination of knowledge, especially in regional activities.

Some countries in the region may graduate from or not request additional HNP lending (e.g., China). In some countries whose agenda for the HNP sector is unfinished, maintaining oversight of HNP issues will be important as part of the overall country strategy (CAS/CDF). In some cases, HNP issues may be addressed in multisectoral programs that are likely to involve human development issues (e.g., urban poverty).

The region also includes a large set of countries with poor health outcomes and less-developed health systems: Cambodia, Lao PDR, Myanmar, North Korea, some Pacific Islands, and Papua New Guinea. Here, drawing on lessons learned from earlier projects in the region will be important. This group will also be a primary target for analytic and advisory services.

The last group of countries—Indonesia, the Philippines, and Vietnam—comprises the largest volume in the portfolio. With their relatively developed health systems, these countries have made important progress in health outcomes but have an important unfinished agenda in the strategy's key priority areas. Bank assistance is likely to focus on evaluation and implementation of key policy reforms and choices such as health financing reforms, regulation, capacity building, and decentralization. This will require more piloting, analytic work, and use of a more diverse set of lending instruments.

Improving Portfolio Quality

Recent assessments of the HNP portfolio indicate mixed success in implementation. It is critical to stress portfolio quality and put in place the needed quality assurance processes.

Improving portfolio quality is likely to require: strengthening the monitoring capacity in both Bank operations and the client countries; improving linkages between analytic work and the lending program; better adapting and using lending instruments to better

---

Box 3-1. Lessons from World Bank Experience in HNP Development Effectiveness

According to a recent appraisal of the Bank's work in health, nutrition, and population, the Bank has been more effective in expanding service delivery than in improving quality and efficiency or furthering institutional change in the past 30 years. The study, by the Operations Evaluation Department, found that during implementation the Bank has generally focused more on providing input than on monitoring outcomes and has not paid enough attention to determinants of health outside the health care system. Promoting health sector reforms, OED said, is likely to require more flexible instruments that could emphasize learning and knowledge transfer. These factors apply (with varying degrees) to the EAP portfolio. OED recommended that to improve the effectiveness of the HNP portfolio the Bank should:

• Enhance quality assurance and results orientation.
• Intensify learning from lending and nonlending services.
• Enhance partnerships and selectivity.

Source: World Bank, 1999b.

address the diverse needs of the sector and the countries; and increasing selectivity in the portfolio. The Bank also needs to strengthen its collaboration with governments to address portfolio implementation issues. This requires closer Bank involvement during supervision and greater emphasis on monitoring and evaluation during project preparation, implementation, and completion.

Quality assurance processes are another key to improving portfolio quality. These processes must take into account the recent changes in the Bank—more decentralized system with more flexible staff arrangements—and the client countries, many of them also going through decentralization. The exact format of the quality assurance process cannot be described here since it must evolve and adapt as portfolio needs change.

Empowering staff is another important dimension of quality. Staffing patterns should reflect the portfolio's size and needs. The unit must address this issue as part of the strategy implementation. Such an exercise should reflect the current skill mix, location of staff, and future needs, after taking into account the sector priorities and needs. Although this exercise is internal, it is critical for the strategy's successful implementation. For instance, much of the policy reform agenda could be best achieved with closer collaboration and regular interaction with the client, one advantage of having a more field-based staff. The region should also ensure that staff has the means to be effective through resource allocations, training and professional development, and support systems.

Ensuring adequate quality also requires backing up Bank initiatives and operations by adequate budget allocations. This may require a shift from annual budget allocations to three- to five-year budget plans, increased flexibility and fungibility of resources, and greater differentiation in resource needs of certain products like pilot projects. Incentives are also needed to foster cross-sectoral collaboration. Although this is one of the Bank's comparative advantages, the current structure does not support cross-sectoral efforts. For instance, devoting more effort and analysis for cross-cutting issues and intersectoral collaboration when preparing country assistance strategies can enhance this.

Improving Client Services

Improving development effectiveness of the Bank's work also requires enhancement of the Bank's services to clients. Client services can be improved by:

- ensuring clients better access to information and HNP databases through a variety of printed and electronic media
- providing more user-friendly documentation to assist the project management team, especially at the local levels
- increasing access to Bank documents in local languages
- working closely with networks and regional management to ensure that Bank processes are responsive to sector and country needs
- using a broader range of lending instruments to respond to the diversity of sector issues
- collaborating more strongly with clients during project implementation
- seeking and using feedback from clients on Bank performance.

Strengthening Partnerships

Effective partnerships with clients, civil society, stakeholders, regional institutions, and other agencies are necessary to address several elements of the strategy. For instance, promoting sector reforms requires understanding stakeholders' interests and formulating coalitions for reform. Similarly, cross-sectoral activities call for work with other partners.

The Bank has been working closely with a number of partners in the region. These include: the Asian Development Bank; UN Agencies (including WHO, UNICEF, UNAIDS, UNFPA, UNDP, UNIDO); bilaterals (European Union, Australian Agency for International Development, DFID, Japan); international NGOs; and foundations (Ford Foundation, Population Council). For example, in Vietnam, the Bank has been working with the government, the UN agencies, and bilateral donors on the development of a health sector strategy. In Indonesia, the Bank has a long-standing and effective collaboration with WHO. The Bank has developed or cofinanced a number of projects with ADB in Cambodia, Laos, and Papua New Guinea. The Population Council has worked closely with the Bank in developing the reproductive health agenda. In addition, many research institutes (e.g., in Hong Kong and Singapore) have participated in Bank analytic work. The strategy calls for strengthening and fostering these partnerships.

This paper cannot list all of the many examples collaboration with other partners, including knowledge production and management of technical issues, lending operations, and analysis. As noted earlier, the CDF exercise that has started in some countries provides a good framework for strengthening such efforts

Implementation Issues

Implementing the strategy will have direct implications for the content of the HNP program in the EAP region. The exact nature of the work program implications will be worked out at country level. The Strategy Matrix illustrates the implication of the strategy for the content of the Bank's work in the HNP sector (Annex A). These implications are summarized below.

Policy advice and assistance strategies. Addressing the sector priorities requires strengthening the CAS/CDF process in the following areas: analysis and linkages between HNP issues and macro-economic issues; linkages and policy coordination in multisectoral issues that affect the HNP sector; and providing a framework for addressing institutional issues and issues that may go beyond the sector but affect its capacity and performance. The CDF exercise could also facilitate partnerships and coordination with other donors and stakeholders.

Lending operations. Although the current portfolio is consistent with current priorities, some high-priority areas have not received adequate attention. The current strategy calls for increased emphasis on such priority areas, depending on their relevance to specific country needs. Moreover, the strategy calls for more flexibility and diversity in the type of lending instruments the HNP sector uses, instruments that are more responsive to sector needs in the different countries. In addition, the strategic direction set in this paper calls for more use of pilot projects as stand-alone products or within investment projects with strong evaluation components. This in turn will require alternative approaches for the management and supervision of such pilot projects.[11] Some of these

topics are illustrated in the Strategy Matrix and include targeting the poor, alternative incentive structure for delivering basic health services to the poor, improving demand for health services, and social insurance programs (Annex A). Another challenge for the HNP sector in the EAP region is the "mismatch" between the complexity of the issues facing the sector and the generally weak institutional capacity of ministries of health to deal them. Many HNP capacity-building efforts have had limited effects because they have focused on only part of the problem (e.g., skill shortages) and not on the more complicated issues of public sector management and performance. Improving the Bank's role in capacity-building efforts will require a better understanding of institutional issues and design and implementation of capacity-building projects or project components. This critical part is essential to ensure sustainability of HNP investments.

Analytic and advisory services (AAA). Sharpening the Bank's strategic direction is likely to require more focused investments in producing and disseminating analysis and providing technical assistance to client countries. At present, knowledge about many of these areas is, at best, incomplete. Analytic work at the country level and selected efforts at the regional level must be given more attention.

- *Analytic work at country level.* At the country level, developing HNP strategies that take a medium- to long-term perspective of the sector is a high priority. In addition, key priority issues require analytic work—such as analysis of health outcomes by poverty, assessing the overall performance of the health care system (both public and private), and analysis of health financing issues. The exact activities will be formulated at the country level, but priority should be given to activities that are closely linked with the lending program or key policy issues that affect the sector's performance.

- *Analytic work at regional level.* A relatively neglected area is analytic work at the regional level. The EAP region, rich and diverse, offers many useful insights and lessons. Among the areas that may require further analysis at the regional level are health promotion and demand programs, approaches to building institutional capacity for health programs (especially policy and regulation), lessons learned from health financing and social insurance efforts, and relationships between the public and the private sectors.

- *Knowledge management.* Managing the knowledge generated through analytic work and operations is an important element in implementing the strategy, which has not received adequate attention in the past. This would require more participation in the generation of knowledge, diversification of products through which knowledge is disseminated, and better utilization of information technology.

The above discussion illustrates a number of direct implications of the strategy on the HNP program in the EAP region. However, to make the strategy effective, it is also important to focus on how it will be integrated into the region's work program to produce the desired results. This is likely to involve:

- using the strategy to guide regular review process of Bank products (both lending and AAA activities) and as a tool for setting priorities
- ensuring consistency between the regional strategy and the country-specific strategies
- monitoring the integration of the Strategy in CAS and CDF efforts in the region and progress in addressing multisectoral issues affecting HNP outcomes
- using the strategy as a guide for Bank-wide monitoring and evaluation activities such as those carried out by the Quality Assurance Groups or the Bank's Operations Evaluation Department

- using strategy development to guide future staffing needs for the unit, including skill mix and staff location
- updating the strategy regularly to ensure that any developments in the sector and the region are taken into account (see below)
- utilizing the strategy to strengthen partnerships in the region.

The EAP HNP Strategy—An Ongoing and Dynamic Process

The strategy development process will be ongoing and dynamic, building on best practices and experiences within the region and internationally. This paper is a first step toward that objective. The next steps would involve consultation with clients and partners in the region, which should not be limited to discussing the strategy paper but should be an ongoing process for sharing knowledge and information across countries and projects.

Implementation of the strategy should also be monitored closely. This will assist the Bank in strengthening its strategic focus and will identify any pitfalls to its implementation. Periodically, sector assistance strategy updates will be needed (these could follow the CAS update format and could be biannual). These updates should take into account discussions and feedback from client countries, Bank management, new developments in the sector, and consultations with other partners. The process of preparing such updates will also encourage greater dissemination of HNP issues and facilitate stronger partnerships.

Notes

1. In addition to persistent income differentials, there is also substantial regional variation in health outcomes and service utilization in most countries of the region. In Indonesia, for example, the U5MR during the period 1992–97 was above 80 per 1,000 live births in 5 of 27 provinces, while it was under 40 per 1,000 in 4 other provinces. In addition to the obstacles associated with poverty (due in part to the fact that most recent gains in agricultural productivity have been confined to irrigated areas), regional variation in health gains may reflect physical barriers to the provision of health services (mountainous terrains, low population density) or linguistic and cultural barriers (e.g., ethnic minorities in Vietnam).

2. Moderate anemia, or iron deficiency, is defined as a hemoglobin level of less than 11 grams per deciliter.

3. The situation with TB treatment in the region provides a good example of the dangers. According to a recent study many persons infected with TB in urban areas of Indonesia and the Philippines treat themselves with drugs purchased over-the-counter at pharmacies (Pathania 1998). Even if they seek care from private providers, there is little attempt to follow up clients, many of whom drop out before the disease has been controlled.

4. For example, part of the strategy can be phased randomly into geographic areas in such a way as to meet the requirements of a controlled experiment (Newman, Rawlings, and Gertler 1994).

5. Government health workers are not permitted to have private practices in Malaysia. However, it is very common in Indonesia.

6. Among the countries in the region, Malaysia has decentralized successfully. The experience of China and the Philippines with decentralization has been less satisfactory. Indonesia will go through a major decentralization exercise during the next two years.

7. Although community financing worked during the period of cooperative agriculture, reforms introduced in the late 1980s deprived commune health centers of their secure source of income. In 1993, the government recentralized the system to some extent by making some commune health center workers in each commune paid civil servants.

8. It is also somewhat limited by the governments' tendency to subsidize inpatient care in government hospitals, since this reduces the risk of catastrophic health care costs and therefore the demand for insurance.

9. In China, rural health insurance coverage was as high as 85 percent in 1975 before economic reforms began to undermine the system of agricultural collectives that used to finance the Cooperative Medical System (CMS). Today, rural insurance coverage in China is only about 10 percent.

10. Singapore introduced mandatory medical savings accounts in 1984. The amount of undisbursed funds accumulated in members' accounts is already enough to finance four years of the country's total health expenditure (World Bank 1998a).

11. At present, there is no differentiation in the supervision of pilot programs and regular investment lending.

References

Ainsworth, Martha; L. Fransen; and M. Over (eds.). 1998. *Confronting AIDs: Evidence from the Developing World.* European Community. Brussels.

Asian Development Bank. 1999. *Policy for the Health Sector.* Publication # 090499. Manila, February.

Economic and Social Commission for Asia and the Pacific. 1998. ESCAP Population Data Sheet. Bangkok.

Economist Intelligence Unit. 1998. "Country Profile— Malaysian Healthcare: The Slow Road to Privatization." Hong Kong.

Fauci, A. 1999. "The AIDS Epidemic: Considerations for the 21st Century." *New England Journal of Medicine 341*(14): 1046–50.

Frankenberg, E. D. Thomas; and K. Beegle. 1999. "The Real Costs of Indonesia's Economic Crisis: Preliminary Findings from the Indonesia Family Life Surveys." Santa Monica, Calif.: RAND. Processed.

Hong, P. K. and Y. M. Teng. 1997. "Health Care Financing in Old Age: Singapore Case Study." Paper presented at the Conference on Financing Health Care and Old Age Security, Singapore, November 8, Institute of Policy Studies/World Bank.

Gong, Y. L., J. P. Koplan; W. Feng; C. H. Chen; P. Zheng; and J. R. Harris. 1995. "Cigarette Smoking in China: Prevalence, Characteristics and Attitudes in Minhang District." *Journal of the American Medical Association 274:* 1232-34.

Gwatkin, D. R., and M. Guillot. 1998. "The Burden of Disease among the Global Poor: Current Situation, Future Trends, and Implications for Research and Policy." Paper prepared for the Global Forum for Health Research, Washington, June.

International Road Federation. 1998. World Road Statistics. Geneva: IRF.

Jin, S. G., Bao-Yu, Lu, and Wei, Li. 1988. "An Evaluation on Smoking-Induced Health Costs in China." Biomedical and Environmental Sciences 8: 342–49.

Lieberman, Samuel. 1999. "Indonesia's Health Strategy Before and After the Crisis." Draft. Jakarta: World Bank. Processed.

Macro International, Inc. Various years. Demographic and Health Surveys (DHS). Calverton, Md.: Macro International.

Murray, C. and A. Lopez. 1996. *Health Dimensions of Sex and Reproduction.* Global Burden of Disease and Injury Series. Geneva: World Health Organization.

Newman, J.; L. Rawlings; and P. Gertler. 1994. "Using Randomized Control Designs in Evaluating Social Sector Programs in Developing Countries." *The World Bank Research Observer 9*(2): 181–201.

Peto R; A. D. Lopez; J. Boreham; M. Thun; and C. J. Heath. 1994. *Mortality from Smoking in Developed Countries 1950–2000: Indirect Estimates from National Vital Statistics.* Oxford: Oxford University Press.

_____. 1992. "Mortality from Tobacco in Developed Countries: Indirect Estimation from National Vital Statistics." *Lancet* 339: 1268-78.

Pathania, Vikram S. 1998. "The Role of the Private Health Sector in Tuberculosis Control and Feasible Intervention Options (with a focus on East Asia and the Pacific Region)." Submitted to HNP Unit of EAP (July). Washington: World Bank.

Poppele, J.; S. Sumarto; and L. Pritchett. 1999. "Social Impacts of the Indonesian Crisis: New Data and Policy Implications." Draft report (May 17). Washington: World Bank.

Prescott, N. 1998. "Health Policy Reform in East Asia." Presentation at the World Bank, East Asia and Pacific Health Sector meeting, September 23, Manila.

Saadah, F.; H. Waters; and P. Heywood. 1999. "Indonesia, Undernutrition in Young Children." Watching Brief. East Asia and Pacific Region, no. 1.

Saadah F. and M. Pradhan. 1999. "Health Care during Financial Crisis: What Can We Learn from the Indonesian National Socioeconomic Survey". The World Bank. East Asia and Pacific Region. Washington.

South Pacific Commission. 1999. Pacific Island Population Data Sheet. Noumea, New Caledonia: SPC.

UNAIDS [Joint United Nations Program on HIV/AIDS] and World Health Organization. 1998. Report on the Global HIV/AIDS Epidemic. Geneva: UNAIDS/WHO, June.

UNICEF/WHO. 1996. *Revised Estimate of Maternal Mortality: A New Approach.* New York: UNICEF/WHO.

UNICEF. 1999. *State of the World's Children.* New York: UNICEF.

United Nations, Population Division. 1999. World Population Prospects: The 1998 Revision. New York: UN.

United Nations, Statistics Division. Quarterly. Population and Vital Statistics Report. New York: UN.

Westinghouse Health Systems. 1985. Malaysia Health Services Financing Study. Final report to the Asian Development Bank. Kuala Lumpur: Asian Development Bank/Westinghouse Overseas Service Corp.

World Bank. 1999e. Confronting AIDs: Public Priorities in a Global Epidemic. Washington.

_____. 1999d. Intensifying Action Against HIV/AIDs in Africa. Washington.

_____. 1999c. Investing in Health: Development Effectiveness in Health, Nutrition, and Population. Washington: Operations Evaluation Department.

_____. 1999b. Curbing the Epidemic: Governments and the Economics of Tobacco Control. Washington: Human Development Network.

_____. 1999a. Population and the World Bank: Adapting to Change. Washington: Human Development Network.

_____. 1998d. "Vietnam Health Sector and Expenditure Review: Concept Note." Washington. Processed.

_____. 1998c. "Samoa Health Sector Review, Meeting the Challenge of Development." Washington: EASHN Department.

_____. 1998b. "Republic of the Philippines: Health, Nutrition and Population Strategy Note." Washington: EASHN Department. Processed.

_____. 1998a. "Health Policy Reform in East Asia." Washington: Health Sector Unit, East Asia Region. Processed

_____. 1997. Sector Strategy: Health, Nutrition and Population. Washington.

_____. 1996. China: Issues and Options in Health Financing, report no. 15278-CHA. Washington: China and Mongolia Department, Human Development Department.

_____. 1994b. Health Priorities and Options in the World Bank's Pacific Member Countries. Washington.

———. 1994a. Indonesia's Health Workforce: Issues and Options, report no. 12835. Washington.

World Health Organization. Various years. World Health Statistics Annual. Geneva.

———. 1999c. Malaria, 1982-1997. *Weekly Epidemiological Record*, 74 (265-272). Geneva.

———. 1999b. *Weekly Epidemiological Record*, June. Geneva.

———. 1999a. Global Tuberculosis Control: WHO Report. Geneva.

———. 1997. Tobacco or Health: A global status report. Geneva.

———. 1996. TB/HIV: A Clinical Manual. Global Tuberculosis Programme. Geneva.

WHO and UNICEF. 1996. Revised Estimates of Maternal Mortality: A New Approach by WHO and UNICEF. Geneva.

WHO/UNICEF/IVACG Task Force. 1997. *Vitamin A Supplements: A Guide to Their Use in the Treatment and Prevention of Vitamin A Deficiency and Xerophthalmia*, second edition. Geneva: World Health Organization.

Annex A. East Asia and Pacific Health, Nutrition, and Population Sector Matrix (FY 00-04)

Underlying HNP issues	Development objectives	EAP's HNP Strategy	Bank instruments		Progress indicators
			Loans/credits	Advisory and analytic activities	
Health, nutrition, and population (HNP) outcomes for poor are lagging. Factors contributing to this discrepancy include: uneven progress in addressing key public health problems among countries, and inequitable use of key public health interventions by poor and other vulnerable groups.	*Improve HNP outcomes of poor by:*	The EAP HNP Strategy will include:	Lending program would support efforts to:	Analysis of health differentials for the poor and nonpoor for different countries to include:	The following indicators should be monitored subnationally and nationally as well as among poor and vulnerable groups:
	Promoting and sustaining cost-effective public health interventions	Ensuring use of efficient, equitable, and sustainable approaches to provide cost-effective interventions to address key public health problems of poor in every country	Increase portfolio targeting and selectivity in terms of programs supported, giving priority to cost-effective public health interventions and public goods	Cost-effectiveness analysis of various public health interventions	*Health Indicators* • Infant and child mortality • TB incidence • HIV/AIDS prevalence *Nutrition Indicators* • Child malnutrition (stunting) • Maternal anemia
	Addressing inequalities in use of key public health interventions	Developing special approaches, as needed, to raise public health service use rates of poor and other vulnerable groups	Improve targeting of government subsidies to poor, in conjunction with sector reform efforts, where applicable	Benefit-incidence analysis of different programs and health care services	Maternal and Reproductive Health • Fertility levels • Adolescent fertility
			Address key constraints to service use by poor, especially quality of services	Analysis of determinants of health service use by the poor and the system's ability to target the poor	*Health Care Services* • Immunization coverage • Professionally attended births • Improved benefit incidence of public sector funding
			Use pilot program to test innovative approaches to better reach the poor	Evaluation of innovative approaches to reach the poor	
	Maintaining policy oversight in intersectoral areas that most affect poor	Working with other sectors to promote healthy intersectoral policies in areas that most affect poor: environment, water and sanitation, school health, and credit programs.	Strengthen collaboration with other sectors through joint or coordinated lending initiatives	Joint analytic and advisory activities	
			Use pilot programs to test innovative approaches for addressing multisectoral approaches to improve health outcomes of the poor	Evaluation of innovative approaches to address multisectoral approaches to improve health outcomes of the poor	

Bank instruments

Underlying HNP issues	Development objectives	EAP's HNP Strategy	Loans/credits	Advisory and analytic activities	Progress indicators
Low performance of health care system as evidenced by high prevalence of unhealthy practices and behaviors; wasteful and ineffective spending on private services; weak capacity of ministries of health in critical nonservice delivery functions, especially policy analysis; inefficient and inequitable government health care delivery systems; poor-quality health care services; inadequately regulated private sector; and inadequate integration of private sector into public health and social insurance programs.	*Enhance performance of health care systems by:*	The strategy will consist of:			Consumer Behavior • Smoking prevalence • Percent of population self-treating illnesses • Percent of private health expenditures spent on drugs • Number of drugs prescribed per outpatient visit • Nutritional knowledge
	Strengthening consumer knowledge of health risks and ability to make informed choices in health care markets.	Developing effective consumer education and health promotion programs	Support programs that provide consumer education and information and empower consumer as a stakeholder in delivery of health care services	Doing comparative studies of efforts to empower and inform consumers and provide effective health promotion programs	
	Strengthening institutional capacity of health ministries in areas of regulations, quality control, consumer education, policy analysis, monitoring, and evaluation	Increasing ministry of health capacity to regulate and control quality, educate consumers, analyze policy, and monitor and evaluate health programs	Address capacity-building needs of ministries of health in nonservice delivery areas through project components or stand-alone lending.	Doing comparative studies of efforts to strengthen capacity of ministries of health to conduct policy analysis, regulatory and quality control functions, consumer education, monitoring and evaluation.	*Capacity of Ministries of Health* (additional indicators needed for measuring capacity of ministry of health in areas of regulation, quality control, consumer education, policy analysis, and monitoring and evaluation)
	Improving performance of public health system	Improving efficiency and equity of government health systems by modifying incentives and pricing Improving implementation of decentralization policies	Test feasibility and potential impact of alternative incentives and pricing policies with pilot programs and research studies Assist governments in preparing and implementing decentralization	Evaluating and disseminating results of pilot programs to test feasibility of alternative incentives and pricing policies Disseminating lessons learned about decentralization and its potential impact on health services	*Efficiency and Equity of Government Health Systems* • Quality of care • Technical efficiency (e.g., productivity per health worker, hospital beds/occupancy ratio) • Allocative efficiency (e.g., percent of total recurrent health budget absorbed by salaries) • Share of government subsidies captured by poorest quintile
	Mobilizing private sector resources to participate in public health and social insurance programs	Involving private sector in providing services for poor by demand-side financing and contracting out curative services to private sector Including private providers in social insurance programs	Include private sector in health programs and pilot feasibility of demand-side financing	Evaluating and disseminating results of pilots to test feasibility of demand-side financing.	*Private Sector* • Quality of care • Percent of public health services received from private sector • Percent of social insurance payments received by private sector • Others
	Supporting new approaches and technologies for disease control	Implementing cost-effective new approaches for disease control and technologies for improving health care systems	Support inclusion of cost-effective new approaches and technologies in Bank supported programs	Conducting economic and technical assessments of new approaches and technologies	*New Approaches/Technologies* • Cost-effective new approaches to addressing key public health concerns

Bank instruments

Underlying HNP issues	Development objectives	EAP's HNP Strategy	Loans/credits	Advisory and analytic activities	Progress indicators
Financing of health care is inadequate or unsustainable. This is illustrated by:	*Secure sustainable health care financing by:*				*Financing*
• Relatively low spending on health	Securing adequate financing, especially for priority programs and increased efficiency in allocating resources	Increasing government spending on health	Address health financing issues in SAL lending operations, where appropriate	Monitoring and reporting health expenditures by key indicators	• Government health spending as percent of GDP
• Relatively low share of government spending directed to public health services					• Percent of government health spending directed to public health services
• High share of spending financed by out-of-pocket expenditures		Reallocating resources from curative outpatient services to priority public health programs	Improve targeting of government funding through health sector reform programs		• Percent of total health spending financed from off-budget sources
• Relatively little use of off-budget sources of funding	Expanding access to sustainable risk pooling	Expanding social insurance coverage, particularly in rural areas and among urban informal sector workers	Support pilot programs to test social insurance models	Doing analysis and evaluation of social insurance programs and pilots	*Risk Pooling*
• Low coverage of health insurance and other risk-pooling services for catastrophic care costs			Support expansion of social insurance programs that are have been evaluated and proven effective		• Percent of population covered by social insurance
• Lack of progress in extending social insurance coverage to rural and urban informal sector workers					• Percent of poor and vulnerable groups covered by social insurance
• Inadequate cost control mechanisms built into existing social insurance programs		Building effective cost control mechanisms into social insurance programs	Ensure that design of social insurance programs has built-in mechanisms for cost control	Evaluating cost control measures in region's social insurance programs and disseminating results	• Percent of inpatient care expenditures covered by social insurance
• Absence of programs like medical savings accounts to support sustainability of social insurance programs with aging population		Developing programs like medical saving accounts to help sustain social insurance programs	Include pilot efforts to address sustainability issues of social insurance programs	Evaluating pilots addressing sustainability of social insurance programs	• Cost control (e.g., average length of stay)
					• Percent of population covered by medical savings account
					• Percent of health care expenditures financed out of pocket

Annex B. Health, Nutrition, and Population Indicators

The Role and Limitations of the Indicators

The indicators shown in the following tables are quantitative measures of countries' health systems and health finance, of their population's health status, and of future issues in health. These indicators provide information on inputs (i.e., how much a country is spending on health), on process and intermediate outcomes (i.e., what proportion of children has been immunized), and on impact (i.e., how much mortality has changed). The main purpose of these indicators is to document the findings of chapters 1 and 2 of this report.

The data must be interpreted with caution, as comparability is often limited because of incomplete data collection, differences in concepts, and use of data from different years. Some of the main limitations concern:

- Mortality indicators, such as life expectancy and infant and child mortality, which are not generally based on accurate vital registration, but are more commonly derived from survey questions, extrapolations with model life tables, and adjustments applied to incomplete measurements. Few countries in the East Asia and Pacific (EAP) Region have complete vital registration, as is shown in Table B-1.
- Disease- and cause-specific indicators are often unreliable because of inadequate surveillance (malaria incidence), relative infrequency of the condition (HIV prevalence and maternal mortality), or adjustments in response to expert opinion, based on incomplete information (tuberculosis estimates).
- Many indicators are based on surveys several years old and have sampling errors that are not shown.

Examples are child malnutrition, contraceptive prevalence rates, smoking prevalence, and immunization coverage.

- Some indicators are estimates provided by country programs or ministries, many of which have inadequate monitoring systems. Immunization coverage of children, for example, is frequently shown to be much lower in well-conducted health surveys than in program statistics.
- Health expenditure data for countries without national health accounting systems (most countries in the EAP region) are based on a combination of government budget estimates of public expenditures, household expenditure surveys for out-of-pocket expenses, and insurance publication and international donor data. Frequently, public expenditures by provinces and states are incomplete, and private expenditures are subject to substantial measurement errors.

Despite these limitations, the indicators shown in the tables will assist in implementing and monitoring the strategy by:

- identifying countries that have and have not made rapid progress in reducing mortality and morbidity among vulnerable groups (i.e., infants, children, and women)
- recognizing the importance of different conditions and diseases: In which countries does malnutrition contribute to ill health? Where are high fertility and reproductive health issues most pressing?
- identifying future challenges: Which countries have rapidly aging populations? Where will emerging

diseases such as HIV strike hardest? Where is public spending high while outcomes are poor?

HNP-at-a-Glance (Tables B-2 and B-3)

Tables B-2 and B-3 show a limited set of indicators (also included in the tables that follow) that give a "snapshot" of the health status and health systems of the countries in the EAP region. Indicators are shaded when their level is worse than the mean of low- and middle-income countries globally, illustrating which countries and which indicators present the biggest challenges.

Selected Findings from the Tables

This section highlights key findings from the tables. For some countries and indicators, the data in the annex tables may differ from those in the main text. The data in the annex tables have used standardized definitions and reference periods, whereas data shown in the main text are at times drawn from specific surveys using different samples and definitions.

Health Status: Morbidity and Mortality
(Tables B-4–B-6)
The decline in mortality since 1970, the first year shown in the table, has been impressive in every country in the region. Yet some countries have made much more rapid progress in reducing childhood mortality. Overall, "under-5" mortality has declined by more than 60 percent, but it remains above the developing-country average in some countries in the region. Mortality by gender shows substantial progress in women's health status. But survey findings show that in some countries in the region, girls between ages 1 and 5 have higher mortality than boys of the same age group, whereas lower mortality would be expected, indicating unequal access to nutrition, health care, and other household resources.

Tuberculosis incidence in the region is the third highest of all Bank regions (after Sub-Saharan Africa and South Asia). Cambodia has one of the highest levels of any country. HIV/AIDS is emerging as a serious

health issue in some of the region's populations but is still relatively low in many others. Malaria incidence data are shown only to give an impression of where this is a serious issue. The surveillance data are too incomplete to allow a comparison across countries.

Nutrition (Table B-7)
The most common indicator of child malnutrition is weight for age (underweight). Being underweight, even mildly, has long-term consequences for cognitive development and contributes to the risk of dying from a large number of causes. Height for age (stunting) reflects linear growth achieved pre- and postnatally. A deficit indicates cumulative effects of inadequacies of diet and health. Stunting is often considered a proxy for long-term deprivation.

Anemia during pregnancy can harm both the mother and fetus, causing loss of the baby, premature birth, or low birthweight. Low birthweight raises the risk of infant mortality and is associated with slow development. The data are not, however, always reliably measured, and comparisons among countries should not be attempted.

Reproductive Health (Table B-8)
Family planning programs, mostly publicly funded in the EAP region, have been successful in providing contraceptives to couples of reproductive age, resulting in a rapid decline in fertility. In 1970, only one country (Japan) had replacement-level fertility of about two children; currently, fertility is at replacement level for the region as a whole. However, the decline in fertility has not been evenly distributed. Some countries in the region remain at medium to high levels of fertility. Less progress has been made in making motherhood safer. Maternal mortality ratios remain high in many countries in the region.

Health Finance (Tables B-9 and B-10)
In the mid-1990s, health spending in the EAP was the second lowest of all Bank regions, at 1.7 percent of gross domestic product (GDP). As per capita income increases, both overall spending on health as a percentage of GDP, as well as public spending on health, tends to increase. In current international dollars (PPP) Japan spends more than 30 times more than Indonesia

on health. About 50 percent of health spending in the region is private.

Population Growth and Structure
(Tables B-11 and B-12)

About 30 percent of the world's population lives in the EAP region. As a result of the decline in fertility (Table B-8), population growth rates have fallen, and this proportion is projected to decline gradually. Projections show that the population in the EAP region may increase by more than 300 million in the next 20 years, even as growth rates are assumed to keep declining. Because of the momentum built into the young age structures, the average number of births will decline by only a small amount in the next 20 years, from about 31 million now to 26 million, even as fertility is projected to reach replacement levels in all countries in the region.

The structure of the population is gradually aging (as illustrated in the age pyramids). The proportion over age 60 is increasing the most in countries that experience the earliest fertility declines. As the proportion of young dependents declines because of declining fertility, and the proportion of older dependents increases only gradually, the large age group of working-age adults will increase. The age/dependency ratio is projected to decline from 0.52 now to 0.42 around 2015, before it starts to increase. This decline in dependency has been termed a "demographic bonus," which is generally a one-time occurrence.

Table B-1. Sources of Health Sector Information

Country/region	Vital registration at least 90% complete Births	Deaths	Census year of most recent census	Health, demographic, or household survey Year and type of most recent survey
Brunei	X	X	1991	
Cambodia	-	-	1998	Demographic Survey, 1996; Socioeconomic Survey, 1997
China	-	-	1990	Population Survey, 1995; Rural-Urban Household Survey, 1995
Fiji	X	X	1996	
Indonesia	-	-	1990	DHS, 1997; SUSENAS, 1998; Family Life Survey, 1998
Japan	X	X	1995	Socioeconomic Surveys (continuous)
Kiribati	-	-	1995	
Korea, Dem. Rep.	-	-	1993	
Korea, Rep.	-	-	1995	National Household Suvey (continuous)
Lao PDR	-	-	1995	Social Indicator Survey, 1993
Malaysia	X	X	1991	Household Income/Basic Amenities Survey, 1995
Marshall Islands	X	X	1988	
Micronesia, Fed. States	-	-	1994	
Mongolia	-	X	1989	National Income-Expenditure Surveys, 1996
Myanmar	-	-	1983	Household Survey, 1997
Palau	-	-	1995	
Papua New Guinea	-	-	1990	DHS, 1996; Household Survey, 1996
Philippines	-	-	1995	DHS, 1998; Family Income and Expenditure Survey, 1997
Samoa	-	-	1991	
Singapore	X	X	1990	Household Expenditure Surveys
Solomon Islands	-	-	1986	
Thailand	-	-	1990	DHS, 1987; Socioeconomic Surveys (ongoing)
Tonga	-	-	1986	
Vanuatu	-	-	1989	
Vietnam	-	-	1999	DHS, 1997; LSMS, 1998

Table B-2. HNP at-a-Glance: Mortality, Morbidity, and Nutrition
Health Status, East Asia and Pacific Region

Country/region	Mortality			Morbidity			Nutrition	
	IMR 1997	U5MR 1997	Life expect. 1997	TB incid. per 100,000 1997	HIV/AIDS prev. (%) 1997	Malaria cases 1997	Child malnut. % underweight mr. 1992–98	Anemia % of preg.women mr. 1985–95
Brunei	9	11	76	..	..	..	..	..
Cambodia	103	147	54	539	2.40	115,000	38	..
China	32	39	70	113	0.06	26,800	16	52
Fiji	18	24	73	..	..	..	8	..
Indonesia	44	56	65	285	0.05	161,300	30	64
Japan	4	6	80	29	0.01		..	..
Kiribati	60	..	60	..	..	..	..	..
Korea, Dem. Rep.	56	74	63	178	<0.005	..	..	..
Korea, Rep.	9	11	72	142	0.01	1,700	..	..
Lao PDR	98	..	53	167	..	..	40	..
Malaysia	11	14	72	112	0.04	26,600	20	56
Marshall Islands	..	..	..	..	0.62	..	..	..
Micronesia, Fed. States	30	36	67	..	..	..	..	..
Mongolia	52	68	66	205	0.01	..	12	45
Myanmar	79	131	60	171	1.79	112,500	43	58
Palau	..	..	..	..	..	..	..	..
Papua New Guinea	61	82	58	250	0.19	38,100	30	13
Philippines	35	41	68	310	0.06	42,000	30	48
Samoa	22	..	69	..	..	..	..	..
Singapore	4	6	76	48	0.15		..	..
Solomon Islands	23	28	70	..	..	68,100	21	..
Thailand	33	38	69	142	2.23	97,500	19	57
Tonga	22	23	70	..	..	..	..	..
Vanuatu	37	46	65	..	..	6,100	20	..
Vietnam	35	45	68	189	0.22	65,900	45	52
East Asia and Pacific	37	47	69	151	..	..	..	..

mr most recent year available.

Note: Shaded areas indicate that the estimate for the country is higher than the mean for low- and middle-income countries, except for life expectancy, in which case shaded areas indicate country estimates that are lower than the low- and middle-income mean. For malaria, a low-and middle-income average is not available.

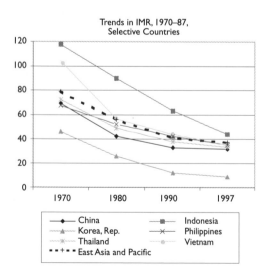

Trends in IMR, 1970–87, Selective Countries

China, Indonesia, Korea, Rep., Philippines, Thailand, Vietnam, East Asia and Pacific

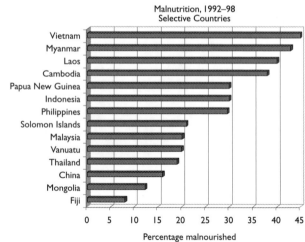

Malnutrition, 1992–98 Selective Countries

Percentage malnourished

Table B-3. HNP at a Glance: Reproductive Health, Immuization, Health Behaviors, and Health Expenditures
Health Status, East Asia and Pacific Region

	Reproductive health			Immunization	Health behaviors		Health expenditures		
		Mat. mort.	Births attended		Smoking prev.		Total, %	Public, %	Per cap.
	TFR	Ratio	by skilled staff	DPT	Male	Female	of GDP	of GDP	US $
Country/region	1997	1990–97	1996–98	1997	1985–95	1985–95	1997 or mr	1997 or mr	1997 or mr
Brunei	2.8	..	..	99	..	..	..	0.8	..
Cambodia	4.6	900	31	70	70	10	7.2	0.7	18
China	1.9	95	85	96	61	7	3.8	2.0	19
Fiji	2.7	..	100	86	..	..	3.4	2.3	69
Indonesia	2.8	390	43	75	53	4	1.8	0.7	17
Japan	1.4	18	..	..	59	15	7.3	5.7	2442
Kiribati	4.2	..	..	91	..	..	..	..	..
Korea, Dem. Rep.	2.0	70	100	..	..	..	..	..	..
Korea, Rep.	1.7	30	95	80	68	7	4.0	2.3	397
Lao PDR	5.6	660	30	60	62	8	2.6	1.3	10
Malaysia	3.2	34	98	91	41	4	2.9	1.4	140
Marshall Islands	..	..	..	78	..	..	..	12.4	..
Micronesia, Fed. States	4.0	..	..	75	..	..	..	..	..
Mongolia	2.6	65	99	92	40	7	4.7	4.3	26
Myanmar	2.4	580	57	90	58	2	..	0.4	..
Palau	..	..	..	91	..	..	..	..	..
Papua New Guinea	4.3	370	53	64	46	28	..	2.8	..
Philippines	3.6	210	56	87	43	8	..	1.3	17
Samoa	4.2	..	52	99	..	..	..	4.9	..
Singapore	1.7	10	100	93	32	3	3.3	1.5	943
Solomon Islands	4.8	..	40	72	..	..	..	3.9	41
Thailand	1.7	200	71	..	49	4	3.9	2.0	96
Tonga	3.6	..	..	95	..	..	..	4.0	..
Vanuatu	4.7	..	50	66	..	..	..	3.3	..
Vietnam	2.4	105	79	87	73	4	5.2	1.1	..
East Asia and Pacific	2.1	..	73	87	59	6	..	..	..

mr, most recent year available.
Note: Shaded areas indicate that the estimate is higher than the mean for low- and middle-income countries (for TFR, maternal mortality ratio, and smoking prevalence, or lower than the mean (for births attended by skilled staff and immunization). Per capita health expenditure is shaded when it falls below $12, the amount needed to buy a minimum package of essential services. Other health expenditure indicators are not shaded.

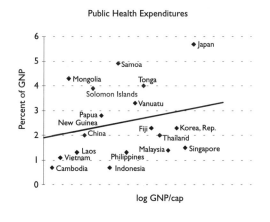

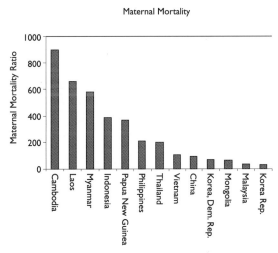

Table B-4. Health Status—Mortality

Country/region	Infant mortality rate				Under-5 mortality rate				Life expectancy at birth			
	1970	1980	1990	1997	1970	1980	1990	1997	1970	1980	1990	1997
Brunei	57	18	9	9	..	..	..	11	67	71	74	76
Cambodia	161	201	122	103	244	330	..	147	42	39	50	54
China	69	42	33	32	120	65	47	39	62	67	69	70
Fiji	49	33	25	18	61	42	31	24	64	68	71	73
Indonesia	118	90	63	44	172	125	83	56	48	55	62	65
Japan	13	8	5	4	21	11	6	6	72	76	79	80
Kiribati	105	..	65	60	..	..	..	..	..	..	57	60
Korea, Dem. Rep.	51	32	45	56	70	43	35	74	60	67	66	63
Korea, Rep.	46	26	12	9	54	18	..	11	60	67	70	72
Lao PDR	146	127	108	98	218	200	..	..	40	45	50	53
Malaysia	45	30	16	11	63	42	21	14	62	67	71	72
Marshall Islands	..	..	..	..	..	..	..	..	..	..	..	..
Micronesia, Fed. States	..	..	39	30	..	..	..	36	..	..	63	67
Mongolia	102	82	63	52	150	..	..	68	53	58	63	66
Myanmar	128	109	94	79	179	134	130	131	49	52	57	60
Palau	..	..	25	..	..	..	34	..	..	..	67	..
Papua New Guinea	112	78	83	61	130	100	..	82	47	51	55	58
Philippines	67	52	42	35	90	81	63	41	57	61	65	68
Samoa	..	..	27	22	..	..	..	..	..	63	66	69
Singapore	20	12	7	4	27	13	8	6	68	71	74	76
Solomon Islands	69	42	29	23	99	56	36	28	..	..	69	70
Thailand	73	49	38	33	102	58	41	38	58	64	68	69
Tonga	..	50	25	22	..	..	27	23	..	..	69	70
Vanuatu	..	..	56	37	..	110	70	46	..	..	61	65
Vietnam	104	57	44	35	157	105	55	45	55	63	67	68
East Asia and Pacific	79	56	41	37	128	83	56	47	59	65	67	69
Europe and Central Asia	..	41	28	23	..	..	35	30	..	68	69	69
Lat. America and Carib.	84	60	41	32	123	..	..	41	61	65	68	70
Middle East/N. Africa	134	95	60	49	200	137	..	63	53	59	65	67
South Asia	139	119	87	77	209	180	..	100	49	54	59	62
Sub-Saharan Africa	137	115	100	91	222	189	..	147	44	48	50	51
High Income	22	13	8	6	28	15	..	7	71	74	76	77
World	98	80	61	56	152	125	..	79	59	63	65	67

Definitions of the indicators

Infant mortality rate: the number of infants who die before reaching 1 year of age, per 1,000 live births in a given year.

Under-5 mortality rate: the probability that a newborn infant will die before reaching age 5, if subject to the age-specific mortality rates for the indicated year.

Life expectancy at birth: the number of years a newborn infant would live if prevailing age-specific mortality rates were to stay at the same level as in the indicated year throughout its life.

Main data sources

Infant mortality rate, under-5 mortality rate, and life expectancy at birth: UNICEF, United Nations Statistics Division, UN Population Division, country statistical offices, and South Pacific Commission

Table B-5. Mortality by Gender

Country/region	Life expectancy at birth								Child mortality rate	
	Males				Females				Males	Females
	1970	1980	1990	1997	1970	1980	1990	1997	Most recent	1988–98
Brunei	63	69	72	73	65	73	77	78	..	..
Cambodia	42	37	49	53	44	40	52	55	..	..
China	61	65	67	68	62	68	70	71	10	11
Fiji	62	66	69	70	65	70	73	75	..	..
Indonesia	47	53	60	63	49	56	63	67	30	27
Japan	69	73	76	77	75	79	82	83	1	1
Kiribati	..	..	54	58	..	..	59	63	..	..
Korea, Dem. Rep.	58	64	64	61	62	70	69	65	..	..
Korea, Rep.	58	64	67	69	62	70	74	76	..	..
Lao PDR	39	43	49	52	42	46	51	55	..	..
Malaysia	60	65	68	70	63	69	73	75	4	4
Marshall Islands	..	..	..	..	..	..	..	..	..	..
Micronesia, Fed. States	..	..	61	65	..	..	65	69	..	..
Mongolia	51	56	61	64	54	59	64	67	..	..
Myanmar	47	50	55	59	50	54	58	62	..	..
Palau	..	..	64	69	..	..	70	73	..	..
Papua New Guinea	47	50	54	57	46	51	56	59	28	21
Philippines	56	59	63	67	59	63	67	70	28	25
Samoa	..	62	64	68	..	64	68	71	..	..
Singapore	65	69	72	74	70	74	77	79	..	..
Solomon Islands	..	..	66	68	..	..	70	73	..	..
Thailand	57	62	66	66	61	67	71	72	11	11
Tonga	..	..	67	69	..	..	71	73	..	..
Vanuatu	..	..	60	63	..	..	62	66	..	..
Vietnam	53	61	64	66	56	65	69	71	11	13
East Asia and Pacific	58	63	66	67	60	66	69	70	..	..
Europe and Central Asia	..	63	65	64	..	72	74	73	..	..
Lat. America and Carib.	58	62	65	66	63	68	71	73	..	..
Middle East and N. Africa	52	57	63	66	54	60	66	68	..	..
South Asia	50	54	59	62	48	54	59	63	..	..
Sub-Saharan Africa	43	46	49	49	46	49	52	52	..	..
High Income	68	70	73	74	74	77	79	80	..	..
World	57	61	63	65	60	65	68	69	..	..

Definitions of the indicators
Life expectancy at birth: the number of years a newborn infant would live if prevailing age-specific mortality rates were to stay at the same level as in the indicated year throughout its life.
Child mortality rate: the probability of dying between ages 1 and 5.

Main data sources
Life expectancy at birth: UNICEF, United Nations Statistics Division, UN Population Division, country statistical offices, and South Pacific Commisson
Child mortality rates: country vital registration systems, and Demographic and Health Surveys.

Table B-6. Health Status—Morbidity

	Tuberculosis		HIV/AIDS		Malaria
Country/region	Incidence per 100,000 people 1997	Prevalence cases (000s) 1997	Adult HIV prevalence (%) 1997	Prevalence cases 1997	Incidence cases 1997
Brunei	..	..	..	..	..
Cambodia	539	101	2.40	130,000	115,000
China	113	2721	0.06	400,000	26,800
Fiji	..	..	..	..	..
Indonesia	285	1606	0.05	52,000	161,300
Japan	29	48	0.01	6,800	..
Kiribati	..	..	..	..	..
Korea, Dem. Rep.	178	91	<0.005	..	..
Korea, Rep.	142	90	0.01	3,100	1,700
Lao PDR	167	17	..	..	..
Malaysia	112	30	0.04	1,100	26,600
Marshall Islands	..	..	0.62	68,000	..
Micronesia, Fed. States	..	..	..	..	..
Mongolia	205	9	0.01	<100	..
Myanmar	171	163	1.79	440,000	112,500
Palau	..	..	..	..	..
Papua New Guinea	250	30	0.19	4,500	38,100
Philippines	310	481	0.06	24,000	42,000
Samoa	..	..	..	..	..
Singapore	48	2	0.15	3,100	..
Solomon Islands	..	..	..	..	68,100
Thailand	142	180	2.23	780,000	97,500
Tonga	..	..	..	..	..
Vanuatu	..	..	..	..	6,100
Vietnam	189	221	0.22	88,000	65,900
East Asia and Pacific	151	..	0.20	..	..
Europe and Central Asia	75	..	0.09	..	..
Lat. America and Carib.	81	..	0.52	..	..
Middle East and N. Africa	66	..	0.13	..	..
South Asia	193	..	0.50	..	..
Sub-Saharan Africa	267	..	7.40	..	..
High Income	24	..	0.30	..	..
World	136	16146	0.97	..	18,715,600

Definitions of the indicators

Tuberculosis incidence: the estimated number of new tuberculosis cases (all forms) per 100,000 people.

Tuberculosis prevalence: the estimated number of people suffering from tuberculosis in 1997, shown in thousands.

Adult HIV prevalence: the percentage of the population aged 15-49 who are infected with HIV. *HIV/AIDS cases:* the number of people of all ages who are living with HIV/AIDS.

Malaria incidence: the number of reported cases of malaria during 1997. The reported numbers are likely to underestimate the true incidence because surveillance systems often include only cases seen by government health services, and for some countries cover only laboratory-confirmed cases. The figures therefore permit only limited comparison between countries.

Main data sources

Malaria: World Health Organization, 1999b.

HIV/AIDS: UNAIDS, 1998.

Tuberculosis: World Health Organization, 1999a.

Table B-7. Nutrition

Country/region	Child malnutrition % of children under 5		Anemia % of pregnant women 1985–95	Total goiter rate % aged 6–11 1985–97	Consumption of iodized salt % of households 1992–98	Low birthweight babies % of births 1993–98
	weight for age 1992–98	height for age 1992–98				
Brunei	..	..	..	..	..	..
Cambodia	38.0	..	..	12	7	18
China	16.0	31.4	52	20	83	6
Fiji	8.0	3.0	..	..	..	..
Indonesia	30.0	42.2	64	28	62	11
Japan	..	..	..	..	..	6
Kiribati	..	..	..	..	..	..
Korea, Dem. Rep.	..	..	..	..	5	..
Korea, Rep.	..	..	..	..	..	4
Lao PDR	40.0	47.3	..	25	93	18
Malaysia	20.1	..	56	20	..	8
Marshall Islands	..	..	..	..	..	..
Micronesia, Fed. States	..	..	..	..	..	..
Mongolia	12.3	26.4	45	31	62	10
Myanmar	42.9	44.6	58	18	14	16
Palau	..	..	..	..	..	..
Papua New Guinea	30.0	..	13	30	..	23
Philippines	29.6	32.7	48	7	15	11
Samoa	..	..	..	..	..	..
Singapore	..	..	..	..	..	..
Solomon Islands	21.0	27.0	..	..	..	..
Thailand	19.0	6.0	57	4	50	7
Tonga	..	..	..	..	..	..
Vanuatu	20.0	19.0	..	..	..	..
Vietnam	44.9	46.9	52	20	65	17
East Asia and Pacific	..	..	..	20	72	..
Europe and Central Asia	..	..	..	22	25	..
Lat. America and Carib.	..	..	..	11	89	..
Middle East and N. Africa	..	..	..	20	48	..
South Asia	..	..	..	17	65	..
Sub-Saharan Africa	..	..	..	19	61	..
High Income	..	..	..	..	..	..
World	..	..	..	18	..	..

Definitions of the indicators

Child malnutrition, weight for age and height for age: the percentage of children under age 5 whose weight for age and height for age are less than minus two standard deviations from the median for the international reference population.

Prevalence of anemia, or iron deficiency, is defined as hemoglobin levels less than 11 grams per deciliter among pregnant women.

Total goiter rate: the percentage of children aged 6–11 with palpable or visible goiter. This is an indicator of iodine deficiency, which causes brain damage and mental retardation.

Consumption of iodized salt: the percentage of households that use edible salt fortified with iodine.

Low-birthweight babies: newborns weighing less than 2,500 grams.

Main data sources

The data are drawn from the World Health Organization, *World Health Statistics Annual,* the United Nations' *Update on the Nutrition Situation,* and UNICEF's State of the World's Children 1999; updates to these sources have been made where new surveys have become available.

Table B-8. Maternal and Reproductive Health

Country/region	Total Fertility Rate Births per woman				Adolescent fertility rate, births to age 15–19 1997	Maternal mortality ratio per 100,000 live births 1990–97	Contraceptive prevalence rate, % of women 15–49 1990–98
	1970	1980	1990	1997			
Brunei	5.6	4.0	3.2	2.8	..	..	..
Cambodia	5.8	4.7	4.9	4.6	14	900	..
China	5.8	2.5	2.1	1.9	15	95	85
Fiji	4.1	3.5	3.1	2.7	..	..	41
Indonesia	5.5	4.3	3.0	2.8	61	390	57
Japan	2.1	1.8	1.5	1.4	3	18	59
Kiribati	..	4.6	4.0	4.2	..	..	..
Korea, Dem. Rep.	6.2	2.8	2.2	2.0	2	70	62
Korea, Rep.	4.3	2.6	1.8	1.7	4	30	79
Lao PDR	6.2	6.7	6.3	5.6	43	660	19
Malaysia	5.5	4.2	3.8	3.2	25	34	48
Marshall Islands	..	..	..	..	..	..	..
Micronesia, Fed. States	..	..	4.8	4.0	..	..	..
Mongolia	5.8	5.3	4.1	2.6	47	65	61
Myanmar	5.8	4.9	3.1	2.4	19	580	17
Palau	..	..	3.1	..	..	..	..
Papua New Guinea	6.1	5.8	5.6	4.3	68	370	26
Philippines	5.7	4.8	4.1	3.6	43	210	48
Samoa	6.7	..	4.8	4.2	..	..	..
Singapore	3.1	1.7	1.9	1.7	10	10	..
Solomon Islands	7.0	6.7	5.6	4.8	..	..	..
Thailand	5.4	3.5	2.2	1.7	70	200	74
Tonga	..	4.8	4.2	3.6	..	..	..
Vanuatu	..	..	5.5	4.7	..	..	..
Vietnam	5.9	5.0	3.6	2.4	28	105	75
East Asia and Pacific	5.7	3.1	2.4	2.1	27	..	..
Europe and Central Asia	2.6	2.5	2.3	1.7	38	..	..
Lat. America and Carib.	5.2	4.1	3.1	2.7	75	..	..
Middle East/N. Africa	6.7	6.2	4.7	3.6	52	..	..
South Asia	6.0	5.3	4.1	3.5	119	..	..
Sub-Saharan Africa	6.6	6.6	6.0	5.5	134	..	..
High Income	2.5	1.9	1.8	1.7	26	..	..
World	4.8	3.7	3.1	2.8	70	..	..

Definitions of the indicators

Total fertility rate: the number of children that would be born to a women if she were to live to the end of her childbearing years and bear children in accordance with current age-specific fertility rates.

Adolescent fertility rate: the number of births per 1,000 women aged 15–19.

Maternal mortality ratio: the number of women who die from pregnancy-related causes, per 100,000 live births.

Main data sources

Fertility rates and contraceptive prevalence rates are estimated from demographic and health surveys, vital registration, and are supplemented with model-based estimates. Maternal mortality estimates are from demographic and health surveys, and UNICEF/WHO, 1996.

Table B-9. Health Finance: Health Expenditures as Percent of GDP

Country/region	Total health expenditures (Percent of GDP)									Public health expenditures (Percent of GDP)								
	1990	1991	1992	1993	1994	1995	1996	1997	1998	1990	1991	1992	1993	1994	1995	1996	1997	1998
Brunei	..	..	..	..	..	..	..	..	..	1.6	1.8	1.9	2.2	2.2	0.8	..	..	..
Cambodia	..	..	..	..	7.2	6.5	6.4	7.1	6.9	..	..	0.2	0.2	0.7	0.4	0.5	0.7	0.6
China	2.7	2.7	2.6	2.4	2.4	2.6	2.6	2.7	2.9	1.2	1.1	0.9	0.7	0.7	0.6	0.6	0.7	0.7
Fiji	..	..	3.4	3.9	3.9	3.8	3.9	3.9	4.3	2.0	2.2	2.3	2.6	2.6	2.5	2.6	2.6	2.9
Indonesia	1.2	1.2	1.3	1.2	1.3	1.2	1.3	1.2	1.3	0.6	0.6	0.7	0.7	0.7	0.6	0.6	0.6	0.6
Japan	6.1	6.1	6.3	6.6	6.9	7.2	7.1	7.1	..	4.7	4.8	4.9	5.2	5.4	5.6	5.7	5.7	5.9
Kiribati	..	..	..	..	..	..	..	..	..	7.8	8.4	8.0	7.7	7.4	7.4	11.0	11.6	..
Korea, Dem. Rep.	..	..	..	..	..	..	..	..	..	..	..	..	..	..	..	..	..	..
Korea, Rep.	5.2	5.0	4.8	5.3	5.1	5.1	5.5	5.6	..	2.1	1.9	1.6	2.1	2.0	2.1	2.5	2.5	..
Laos	..	..	2.4	3.0	3.2	3.1	2.6	3.7	2.6	0.0	..	0.5	1.2	1.5	1.8	1.2	2.3	1.2
Malaysia	2.5	2.6	2.6	2.4	2.3	2.2	2.3	2.3	2.4	1.5	1.6	1.6	1.5	1.3	1.3	1.4	1.3	1.3
Marshall Islands	..	..	..	..	..	..	..	..	..	12.9	13.5	14.4	12.2	..	..	..	..	..
Micronesia, Fed. States	..	..	..	..	..	..	..	..	..	..	..	..	..	..	..	..	..	..
Mongolia	6.7	6.8	4.7	..	..	..	..	..	..	6.0	6.3	4.4	4.4	4.4	4.3	..	..	..
Myanmar	..	..	..	..	..	..	..	1.4	..	1.0	1.0	0.8	0.5	0.4	0.4	0.4	0.3	0.2
Palau	..	..	..	..	..	..	..	..	..	..	..	..	..	..	..	..	..	..
Papua New Guinea	..	..	..	..	..	..	..	3.2	..	3.1	2.8	2.4	2.8	2.8	..	..	2.6	..
Philippines	2.9	2.7	2.8	2.9	3.0	3.2	3.3	3.4	3.7	1.5	1.4	1.3	1.4	1.5	1.5	1.6	1.7	1.7
Samoa	..	..	..	..	..	..	..	..	..	3.9	3.7	3.1	3.5	4.4	3.8	3.8	4.4	4.8
Singapore	3.3	3.6	3.6	3.3	3.1	3.3	3.3	3.2	3.2	1.0	1.3	1.2	1.1	1.0	1.2	1.2	1.1	1.1
Solomon Islands	..	5.8	..	..	..	..	..	4.9	..	5.0	5.0	5.5	5.6	5.8	5.4	4.0	4.2	..
Thailand	5.4	5.2	5.3	5.2	5.2	5.0	5.1	6.1	6.2	1.0	1.1	1.2	1.1	1.3	1.3	1.3	1.7	1.7
Tonga	..	..	..	..	..	..	..	..	..	3.7	4.2	4.0	..	..	..	..	..	..
Vanuatu	..	..	..	..	..	..	..	..	..	2.6	2.5	2.6	2.8	..	..	..	..	..
Vietnam	2.9	..	..	5.3	..	..	..	4.3	..	0.9	0.8	1.0	1.2	..	0.2	0.3	0.4	..
East Asia and Pacific	..	..	..	..	..	..	..	..	1.5	1.6	1.6	1.7	..	..	..	..	..	
Europe and Central Asia	..	..	..	..	..	..	..	..	2.9	3.2	3.3	3.6	4.6	4.2	4.0	..	..	
Lat. America and Carib.	..	..	..	..	..	..	..	..	2.8	2.5	2.6	2.7	2.8	..	..	..	..	
Middle East and N. Africa	..	..	..	..	..	..	..	..	2.5	..	..	..	..	..	..	..	..	
South Asia	..	..	..	..	..	..	..	..	1.2	1.1	..	0.8	0.8	0.8	..	..	..	
Sub-Saharan Africa	..	..	..	..	..	..	..	..	2.3	..	..	2.5	..	..	..	..	..	
High Income	..	..	..	..	..	..	..	..	5.3	5.8	6.0	6.1	6.1	6.3	6.4	6.3	..	
World	..	..	..	..	..	..	..	..	4.7	5.2	5.5	5.5	5.7	..	..	..	..	

Definitions of the indicators

Total health expenditures: the sum of public expenditures and private expenditures on health. Public expenditures consist of recurrent and capital spending from government (central and local) budgets, external borrowings and grants (including donations from international agencies and nongovernmental organizations), and social (or compulsory) health insurance funds. Private health expenditures include direct household (out-of-pocket) spending, private insurance, charitable donations, and direct service payments by private corporations.

Main data sources

Health expenditure estimates come from country sources, supplemented by World Bank country and sector studies. Data were also drawn from World Bank public expenditure reviews, the IMF government finance data files, and other studies. Data on private expenditures are largely from household surveys and World Bank poverty assessments and sector studies.

Table B-10. Health Finance: Health Expenditures per Capita

Country/region	Health expenditures per capita — Current US $								Health expenditures per capita — PPP (Current international $)							
	1990	1991	1992	1993	1994	1995	1996	1997	1990	1991	1992	1993	1994	1995	1996	1997
Brunei	..	..	..	..	..	..	..	..	..	..	..	..	..	..	..	..
Cambodia	..	..	..	..	18	..	..	..	..	..	..	..	..	..	..	..
China	12	12	14	19	..	..	..	..	54	61	69	90	..	..	..	..
Fiji	..	..	69	..	..	..	..	..	..	..	120	..	..	..	..	..
Indonesia	12	13	14	16	17	..	..	..	39	42	48	51	54	..	..	..
Japan	1467	1682	1912	2285	2618	2962	2639	2442	1104	1183	1300	1382	1484	1595	1670	..
Kiribati	..	..	..	..	..	..	..	..	..	..	..	..	..	..	..	..
Korea, Dem. Rep.	..	..	..	..	..	..	..	..	..	..	..	..	..	..	..	..
Korea, Rep.	231	260	273	293	330	392	421	397	306	334	366	394	429	477	522	..
Lao PDR	..	..	..	15	..	10	..	..	..	..	..	..	51	31	..	..
Malaysia	..	..	..	81	..	..	140	..	..	..	..	..	211	..	317	..
Marshall Islands	..	..	..	..	..	..	..	..	..	..	..	..	..	..	..	..
Micronesia, Fed. States	..	..	..	..	..	..	..	..	..	..	..	..	..	..	..	..
Mongolia	..	67	26	..	..	..	..	..	136	126	82	..	..	..	..	..
Myanmar	..	..	..	..	..	..	..	..	..	..	..	..	..	..	..	..
Palau	..	..	..	..	..	..	..	..	..	..	..	..	..	..	..	..
Papua New Guinea	..	..	..	..	..	..	..	..	..	..	..	..	..	..	..	..
Philippines	..	17	..	..	..	..	..	..	..	67	..	..	..	..	..	..
Samoa	..	..	..	..	..	..	..	..	..	..	..	..	..	..	..	..
Singapore	457	578	656	681	777	943	..	..	524	629	695	694	733	829	..	..
Solomon Islands	..	41	..	..	..	..	..	..	..	112	..	..	..	..	..	..
Thailand	..	..	102	..	96	..	..	..	..	..	256	..	230	..	..	..
Tonga	..	..	..	..	..	..	..	..	..	..	..	..	..	..	..	..
Vanuatu	..	..	..	..	..	..	..	..	..	..	..	..	..	..	..	..
Vietnam	3	..	..	9	..	..	..	..	..	..	..	63	..	..	..	..
East Asia and Pacific	..	..	..	..	..	..	..	..	..	..	..	..	..	..	..	..
Europe and Central Asia	..	..	..	..	..	..	..	..	..	..	..	..	..	..	..	..
Lat. America and Carib.	..	..	..	..	..	..	..	..	..	..	..	..	..	..	..	..
Middle East and N. Africa	..	..	..	..	..	..	..	..	..	..	..	..	..	..	..	..
South Asia	..	..	..	..	..	..	..	..	..	..	..	..	..	..	..	..
Sub-Saharan Africa	..	..	..	..	..	..	..	..	..	..	..	..	..	..	..	..
High Income	..	..	..	..	..	..	..	..	..	..	..	..	..	..	..	..
World	..	..	..	..	..	..	..	..	..	..	..	..	..	..	..	..

Definitions of the indicators
Total health expenditures: see Table 7 for definition of health expenditures. Per capita health expenditures are shown in US $ at official exchange rates in 1997, and in PPP (purchasing power parity), using 1997 conversion rates collected by the International Comparison Programme coordinated by the United Nations.

Main data sources
See Table B1-8.

Table B-11. Population Growth

Country/region	Total population Estimate (millions) 1980	Total population Estimate (millions) 1999	Total population Projection (millions) 2020	Growth rate Average annual 1980–99	Growth rate Average annual 1999	Growth rate 1990– 2020	Births Average annual (thousands) 1995–99	Births Average annual (thousands) 2020–24	Deaths Average annual (thousands) 1995–99	Deaths Average annual (thousands) 2020–24
Brunei	0.19	0.32	0.43	2.7	2.0	1.4	7	7	1	2
Cambodia	6.5	10.9	15.4	2.7	2.1	1.6	363	333	130	153
China	981.2	1,249.7	1,428.5	1.3	0.9	0.6	20,807	19,618	9,216	13,176
Fiji	0.63	0.84	1.1	1.5	1.6	1.2	18	18	4	7
Indonesia	148.3	207.0	263.9	1.8	1.6	1.2	4,829	4,416	1,540	2,041
Japan	116.8	126.4	123.3	0.4	0.1	-0.1	1,235	1,091	1,016	1,578
Kiribati	0.06	0.09	0.13	2.1	2.3	1.7	3	2	1	1
Korea, Dem. Rep.	17.7	23.4	27.4	1.5	1.0	0.7	482	423	206	260
Korea, Rep.	38.1	46.8	52.7	1.1	0.8	0.6	709	627	291	466
Lao PDR	3.2	5.1	8.0	2.4	2.4	2.2	188	198	66	71
Malaysia	13.8	22.6	30.6	2.6	2.0	1.4	546	530	104	190
Marshall Islands	0.03	0.06	..	3.8	..	..	..	..	..	..
Micronesia, Fed. States	0.1	0.11	0.16	2.5	1.8	1.7	3	3	1	1
Mongolia	1.7	2.6	3.5	2.4	1.5	1.4	59	60	17	21
Myanmar	33.8	44.9	54.1	1.5	1.2	0.9	935	930	414	604
Palau	0.01	0.02	..	2.3	..	..	..	..	..	..
Papua New Guinea	3.1	4.7	6.8	2.2	2.2	1.7	145	137	44	57
Philippines	48.3	76.7	110.5	2.4	2.1	1.7	2,181	1,987	434	617
Samoa	0.16	0.18	0.25	0.7	1.3	1.5	5	4	1	1
Singapore	2.3	3.2	3.8	1.8	1.8	0.7	47	45	17	31
Solomon Islands	0.23	0.43	0.72	3.3	2.9	2.5	14	16	2	3
Thailand	46.7	61.5	70.5	1.5	0.7	0.6	1,009	949	407	627
Tonga	0.09	0.10	0.13	0.3	1.2	1.1	3	2	1	1
Vanuatu	0.12	0.19	0.29	2.5	2.5	2.1	6	6	1	2
Vietnam	53.7	77.5	102.0	1.9	1.3	1.3	1,611	1,724	496	677
East Asia and Pacific	1,359.4	1,790.0	2,124.1	1.4	1.1	0.8	30,903	30,611	25,697	28,140
Europe and Central Asia	425.8	476.0	491.9	0.6	0.2	0.2	6,248	6,247	5,370	5,566
Lat. America and Carib.	360.3	509.8	690.3	1.8	1.7	1.4	11,534	10,996	3,232	4,604
Middle East and N. Africa	174.1	291.9	424.7	2.7	2.1	1.8	7,709	8,201	1,868	2,463
South Asia	902.6	1,331.1	1,752.5	2.0	1.9	1.3	36,588	34,035	11,811	14,618
Sub-Saharan Africa	380.7	643.8	1,105.3	2.8	2.6	2.6	25,219	29,036	9,161	10,829
High Income	826.9	934.4	982.3	0.6	0.3	0.2	11,345	10,922	8,400	10,409
World	4,429.9	5,977.0	7,571.1	1.6	1.4	1.1	131,779	130,768	52,925	66,851

Definitions of the indicators

Total population, 1980, 1999, and 2020: the estimated and projected mid-year, de-facto population, shown in millions. Current (1999) estimates are in most cases extrapolations from the most recent census. Projections for 2020 are made using the cohort-component method.

Population growth rates: the average annual population growth rate, calculated using the exponential endpoint method.

Births and deaths: estimated and projected annual number, calculated by using age-specific fertility and mortality rates and applying these to the estimated and projected age structure of the population.

Main data sources

Demographic data are obtained from country statistical offices, the United Nations Population Division, regional UN Agencies (ESCAP for the East Asia and Pacific region), and the South Pacific Commission.

Table B-12. Population Structure

Country or Region	Under 15 % of total 1995	15 to 64 % of total 1995	65 + 1995	*Population Structure* Under 15 % of total 2020	15 to 64 % of total 2020	65 + 2020
Brunei	34	63	3	22	68	9
Cambodia	43	54	3	31	64	4
China	26	68	6	20	69	11
Fiji	35	61	4	24	68	9
Indonesia	33	62	4	24	69	7
Japan	16	69	15	13	60	27
Kiribati	40	58	2	29	65	5
Korea, Dem. Rep.	27	68	5	21	71	8
Korea, Rep.	23	71	6	18	70	13
Lao PDR	44	52	4	36	61	3
Malaysia	36	60	4	25	68	7
Marshall Islands	..	..	..	..	..	..
Micronesia, Fed. States	39	57	4	28	67	6
Mongolia	39	57	4	25	70	5
Myanmar	32	64	4	25	69	6
Palau	..	..	..	..	..	..
Papua New Guinea	40	58	3	31	64	4
Philippines	38	58	3	27	67	6
Samoa	39	57	4	29	66	5
Singapore	22	71	6	17	69	15
Solomon Islands	45	53	3	33	63	4
Thailand	28	67	5	20	71	9
Tonga	34	61	5	25	68	7
Vanuatu	41	55	4	32	63	5
Vietnam	37	58	5	25	69	6
East Asia and Pacific	28	66	6	21	69	9
Europe and Central Asia	25	65	10	19	68	13
Lat. America and Carib.	34	61	5	24	68	8
Middle East and N. Africa	40	56	4	29	66	5
South Asia	37	59	4	26	68	5
Sub-Saharan Africa	45	52	3	38	59	3
High Income	19	67	13	16	65	19
World	31	62	7	25	66	9

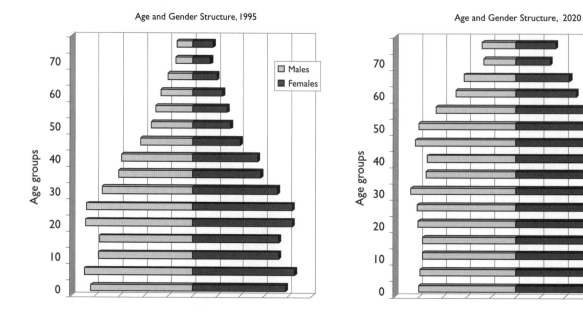

Table B-13. Health System Performance

Country/region	Immunization coverage % of children under age 1		Antenatal care % of women receiving care 1990–98	Tetanus vaccinization % of women 1995–97	Births attended by skilled health staff % of births 1996–98
	Measles 1997	DPT 1997			
Brunei	98	99	100	..	..
Cambodia	68	70	52	..	31
China	96	96	..	..	85
Fiji	75	86	100	100	
Indonesia	71 a	75 a	89	55	43
Japan	..	..	100	100	..
Kiribati	82	91	88	..	..
Korea, Dem. Rep.	..	..	..	100	100
Korea, Rep.	85	80	96	100	95
Lao PDR	67	60	8	32	30
Malaysia	83	91	74	94	98
Marshall Islands	52	78	..	..	..
Micronesia, Fed. States	74	75	90	..	..
Mongolia	98	92	71	..	99
Myanmar	88	90	82	43	57
Palau	83	91	..	..	..
Papua New Guinea	76 a	64 a	77	25	53
Philippines	79 a	87 a	86	77	53
Samoa	99	99	52	..	52
Singapore	89	93	100	100	100
Solomon Islands	68	72	92	..	40
Thailand	92	71	73	96	71
Tonga	97	95	95	..	..
Vanuatu	59	66	98	..	50
Vietnam	77 a	87 a	78	60	79
East Asia and Pacific	93	93	..	36	73
Europe and Central Asia	93	..	..	..	93
Lat. America and Carib.	88	82	..	57	82
Middle East and N. Africa	81	90	..	59	70
South Asia	58	87	..	74	28
Sub-Saharan Africa	..	53	..	39	37
High Income	83	..	..	..	99
World	..	..	..	52	60

Definitions of the indicators

Immunization coverage, measles and DPT: the percentage of children one year of age who have received one dose of measles vaccine, and two or three doses of diphtheria, pertussis, and tetanus (DPT) vaccine.

Pregnant women receiving antenatal care: the percentage of pregnant women who receive pregnancy-related health care provided by a medical professional (doctor, nurse, or midwife).

Pregnant women receiving tetanus vaccination: the percentage of pregnant women who receive two tetanus toxoid injections during their first pregnancy and one booster shot during each subsequent pregnancy.

Births attended by skilled health staff: the percentage of deliveries attended by personnel trained to give the necessary supervision, care, and advice to women during pregnancy, labor, and the postpartum period.

Main data sources

Data on health services are mainly from the WHO's Statistical Information System, which in turn reports data received from national sources. Because country health information systems vary, the data are not always strictly comparable. Immunization data followed by "a" are from demographic and health surveys, which are considered to be more accurate.

Table B-14. Risk Factors

Country/region	Smoking prevalence % of adults Male 1985–95	Female 1985–95	Access to safe water % of population Urban mr, 1990–97	Rural mr, 1990–97	Access to sanitaton % of population Urban 1997 or mr	Rural 1997 or mr	Motor vehicles and traffic accidents Vehicles per 1,000 pop.	People injured/killed 1,000 vehicles
Brunei	..	..	100	92	71	51	..	..
Cambodia	70	10	20	12	..	..	6	31
China	61	7	..	..	68	16	8	22
Fiji	..	..	..	..	..	..	..	
Indonesia	53	4	87	57	88	61	22	1
Japan	59	15	..	..	..	..	547	14
Kiribati	..	..	70	80	83	45	..	..
Korea, Dem. Rep.	..	..	100	100	100	100	..	..
Korea, Rep.	68	7	93	77	100	100	226	34
LaoPDR	62	8	34	36	13	2	4	..
Malaysia	41	4	100	86	94	66	182	14
Marshall Islands	..	..	100	33	88	57	..	..
Micronesia, Fed. States	..	..	..	..	..	..	..	..
Mongolia	40	7	100	68	100	54	28	23
Myanmar	58	2	78	50	56	36	2	..
Palau	..	..	..	..	..	..	..	..
Papua New Guinea	46	28	97	18	95	12	26	..
Philippines	43	8	91	81	88	64	30	2
Samoa	..	..	..	..	100	96	..	..
Singapore	32	3	100	..	100	..	168	14
Solomon Islands	..	..	80	62	60	9	..	..
Thailand	49	4	94	88	98	95	104	13
Tonga	..	..	..	..	..	..	..	..
Vanuatu	..	..	95	75	90	..	..	..
Vietnam	73	4	100	66	..	..	..	..
East Asia and Pacific	59	6	..	..	74	26	16	..
Europe and Central Asia	59	26	..	..	..	..	161	..
Lat. America and Carib.	39	20	83	36	80	40	92	..
Middle East and N. Africa	..	..	98	70	..	..	59	..
South Asia	41	4	84	84	48	9	6	..
Sub-Saharan Africa	..	..	74	32	..	..	21	..
High Income	39	22	..	..	..	..	554	..
World	48	12	..	..	..	..	121	..

Definitions of the indicators

Smoking prevalence: the percentage of men and women aged 15 and over who smoke cigarettes.

Access to safe water: the percentage of the population in urban and rural areas with reasonable access to an adequate amount of safe water (including treated surface water, and untreated, uncontaminated water from springs, and wells).

Access to sanitation: the percentage of the population in urban and rural areas with adequate excreta disposal facilities that can prevent human and animal contact with excreta. Suitable facilities range from simple but protected pit latrines to flush toilets connected to public sewers or household systems.

Traffic accidents: accident-related injuries and deaths reported to the authorities that occur within 30 days of an accident.

Motor vehicles include cars, buses, and freight vehicles.

Main data sources

Data on smoking prevalence are from country surveys. Data on access to safe water and sanitation are from the WHO's EPI Information System: Global Summary, September 1998.

Motor vehicle and traffic accident data are from the International Road Federation, *World Road Statistics 1998.*

Table B-15. Health Services and Personnel

Country/region	Physicians 1990–97	Nurses, midwives per 1,000 population 1990–97	Hospital beds % of pop. 1990–97	Inpatient admissions stay, days 1990–97	Average length of capita 1990–97	Outpatient visits, per 1990–97
Brunei	..	..	..	..	..	..
Cambodia	0.6	1.4	2.1	..	..	..
China	1.1	0.9	2.4	4.2	15.0	..
Fiji	0.4	2.2	..	..	..	..
Indonesia	0.1	0.7	0.7	..	..	..
Japan	1.8	6.4	16.2	8.9	44.0	16.3
Kiribati	0.1	1.9				
Korea, Dem. Rep.	..	..	..	..	..	..
Korea, Rep.	1.2	2.3	4.4	5.7	13.0	10.0
Lao PDR	..	..	2.6	..	..	..
Malaysia	0.4	1.6	2.0	..	..	..
Marshall Islands	..	..	..	..	..	..
Micronesia, Fed. States	0.5	3.3	..	..	..	..
Mongolia	2.7	4.5	11.5	..	..	5.0
Myanmar	0.3	0.4	0.6	..	..	..
Palau	..	..	..	..	..	..
Papua New Guinea	0.2	1.0	4.0	..	..	..
Philippines	0.1	0.4	1.1	..	..	..
Samoa	0.4	1.9	..	..	..	..
Singapore	1.5	4.2	3.6	11.7	..	..
Solomon Islands	..	1.4	..	..	..	..
Thailand	0.2	1.0	1.7	..	..	..
Tonga	..	..	..	..	..	..
Vanuatu	..	..	..	..	..	..
Vietnam	0.4	..	3.8	6.8	7.8	3.3
East Asia and Pacific	..	..	2.1	4.0	15.0	5.0
Europe and Central Asia	..	..	10.1	17.0	14.0	6.0
Lat. America and Carib.	..	..	..	2.0	4.0	2.0
Middle East and N. Africa	..	..	1.8	5.0	8.0	4.0
South Asia	..	..	0.7	..	..	3.0
Sub-Saharan Africa	..	..	1.2	..	..	4.0
High Income	..	..	5.8	14.0	15.0	8.0
World	..	..	3.8	9.0	14.0	6.0

Definitions of the indicators

Physicians: graduates of any faculty or school of medicine who are working in any medical field (practice, teaching, research).

Hospital beds: inpatient beds available in public, private, general, and specialized hospitals and rehabilitation centers. In most cases, beds for both acute and chronic care are included.

Inpatient admission rate: the percentage of the population admitted to hospitals during a year.

Average length of stay: the average duration of inpatient hospital admissions.

Outpatient visits per capita: the number of visits to health care facilities per capita, including repeat visits.

Main data sources

Data on health personnel and use of health services are from the WHO's Statistical Information System, supplemented by country data.

Annex C. The World Bank Role in HNP

Investing in people is at the center of the Bank's work in the EAP region. Investments in health, nutrition, and population are essential components of poverty reduction efforts and are key to sustainable economic growth in the region. Improved health reduces productivity loss; permits the use of natural resources that had been totally or nearly inaccessible because of disease; increases school enrollments and educational attainments; and frees alternative use of resources that would otherwise have been spent on treating illness. Economic gains are greater for poor people who are usually more afflicted by ill health.

Over the past three decades, the Bank has been an important player in the HNP sector in the region through policy advice and dialogue, lending operations, and analytic work. The Bank's level of involvement in the different countries varies significantly, a reflection of the large diversity of issues and needs across the region.

Policy Advice and Assistance Strategies

Country assistance strategies (CAS) are important tools for addressing HNP issues as part of the overall development framework for specific countries. The region has been generally successful in ensuring that HNP issues are highlighted in most CAS exercises. However, the linkages of HNP issues with the macroeconomic analyses and poverty alleviation strategies could be strengthened. In fact, the comprehensive development framework (CDF) provides a great opportunity for achieving this objective. The CDF could also facilitate cross-sectoral efforts needed to address the unfinished HNP agenda.

Bank strategies for the EAP region have emphasized the importance of advisory and consultative services. This involves more involvement of civil societies and professional communities, as well as building partnerships with other multilateral and bilateral agencies. Although many of these activities were intensified during the recent economic crisis, they are likely to remain an integral part of the region's work.

Lending Operations

Since the early 1970s, the Bank has financed HNP programs in 10 countries for a total of $2.2 billion (Figure C-1). Bank financing has been concentrated in China (37 percent) and Indonesia (33 percent). In recent years, the Bank has expanded its support to more countries in the region and is likely to be involved soon in still more of them (e.g., Samoa, Myanmar). The HNP portfolio has grown significantly over the years, especially between 1991 and 1996. However, the last three years (fiscal years 1997, 1998, 1999) saw a decline in the volume of HNP investment lending (the average annual lending reached about a third of the 1996 level). This decline may be partially due to the East Asia financial crisis as well as the graduation of some client countries to IBRD lending terms (e.g., Philippines).[1] Table C-1 summarizes Bank Group HNP operations in 1999.

The EAP contribution to total Bank lending in HNP averaged about 22 percent of total HNP lending between 1993 and 1995. This contribution was reduced to 13 percent in 1996, 7 percent in 1997, and 6 percent in 1998.

EAP human development unit (EASHD) manages about 22 operations with a total lending volume of

Figure C-1.HNP Lending in the EAP Region, Compared to Total HNP Lending in the World Bank, by Year (millions of U.S. dollars)

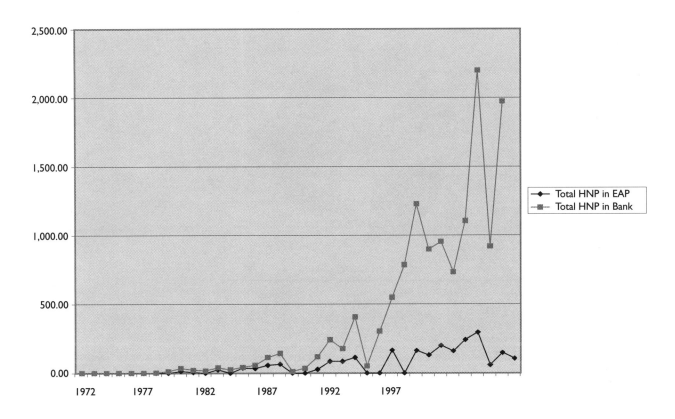

Source: EAP Human Development Sector.

$1.3 billion. About 47 percent of lending volume is in China; 26 percent, in Indonesia (Figure C-2). The distribution of the lending program is especially significant, considering that the future lending program in China is uncertain since its July 1999 graduation from IDA borrowing terms.

In terms of focus, projects cover a wide range of issues, depending on country characteristics (see Strategy Matrix). In general, the Bank finances more "hard ware" components in the region's less developed countries that are still building their health systems. However, the Bank's role has been evolving in other countries, and it has been addressing priority health problems and financing projects to build capacity to make systems run better. China, Indonesia, the Philippines, and Vietnam, fit into this category. In these countries, the Bank has been increasingly financing "software" components of the health care system (e.g., management information systems), approaches to strategic planning, and raising awareness of noncommunicable disease threats. However, many of East Asian countries now face more difficult policy choices related to issues of health workforce, regulation of the private sector, decentralization of health care systems, and targeting of health resources. In response, countries are likely to require assistance that goes beyond scope of the current East Asia Human Development Sector (EASHD) program. To this end, countries may need assistance in designing and implementing more comprehensive policy reform packages. These projects are likely to require a more diverse set of lending instruments such as sector loans and learning and innovation loans [2]

Figure C-2. Distribution of Ongoing HNP Lending Operations in the EAP Region, by Country

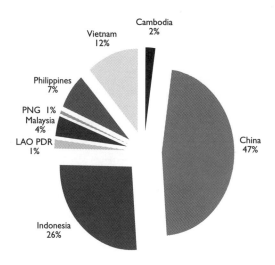

Source: EAP Human Development Sector.

Analytic Work and Technical Assistance

The analytic work (also known as economic sector work—ESW) is an important part of the Bank's work in HNP. ESW is key for policy dialogue and provides the analytic underpinnings of the lending operations. The region has supported ESW that influenced or facilitated important policy changes, has assisted in capacity-building efforts, and has provided the background and analytic basis for important lending operations. The Bank now supports two strategy development exercises in Vietnam and Indonesia. Despite these contributions, the linkages between ESW and lending operations need strengthening.

Analyzing trends in ESW is not easy, given the limitations of the information system(s). Data for the past three years show wide variations in number of products and resources across countries and for the different years. During the past few years, more types of ESW products and or analytic work have been produced. For instance, brief policy and sector notes are regularly used in policy dialogue, and client countries now demand them.

Notes

1.These figures do not include adjustment-lending operations that may involve support for the HNP sector.

2. The major part of the HNP portfolio in EAP relies on sector investment loans (SILs). Recently, the unit has had at least two SILs that are in preparation. In addition, some resources for the HNP sector have been channeled through the SIL prepared in response to the East Asia financial crisis.